TEEN PREGNANCY

Matthew and Lea Dacy
and
Dave Jackson

David C. Cook Publishing Co.
Elgin, Illinois—Weston, Ontario

To our friends in the fight to cherish life.

Special thanks to Becky MacDougall and Sunny Ridge
Family Center, Wheaton, Illinois

David C. Cook Publishing Co.
Elgin, Illinois—Weston, Ontario
Teen Pregnancy
©1989 David C. Cook Publishing Co.

The photographs contained on the cover and throughout this book are stage
dramatizations and are for illustrative purposes only. These photographs do not
depict actual persons engaged in the situations described in this book, nor are
they intended to do so.

Published by David C. Cook Publishing Co.
850 N. Grove Ave., Elgin, IL 60120
Cable address: DCCOOK
Designed by Christopher Patchel and Steve Smith
Photo by Paul Brackley
Illustrated by Jane Sterrett
Printed in the United States of America
Library of Congress Catalog Card Number 88-62829

ISBN: 1-55513-842-X

CONTENTS

INTRODUCTION

Why is a 30-year-old, married man without children writing a book about teenage pregnancy? One reason is that I'm a journalist—a technical writer in the field of health and science. In 1985, there were 9 million females ages 15-19 in the United States. Forty percent of them were sexually active without ever being married. About 980,000 of these young women became pregnant. Roughly half did not carry their children to term: stillbirth and miscarriage played a role, but the overwhelming reason was abortion. Of the 470,000 women who gave birth, 270,000 were unmarried mothers, and 110,000 had given birth at least once before. [1]

Another reason for my interest in this topic is that I'm a Christian. I can report that despite all the grim statistics, teen or crisis pregnancy is a time when God can show remarkable works of grace. I've seen lives transformed.

But the most important reason that I'm writing this book is because of my wife Lea's and my involvement in the Crisis Pregnancy Center in our small, midwestern city. The goal of this center is to offer practical help and spiritual nurture to women in this crisis situation. They may be married or single, teens or older, Christians or unchurched. But they're all in crisis pregnancies and face special needs—medical, financial, emotional.

Lea is part of the staff of this Crisis Pregnancy Center, which opened in 1982, and I am one of the nearly 100 volunteers that help out. The clients who come to these offices represent the complete spectrum of needs related to unwed pregnancy.

Even though Lea and I have not experienced the same kind of trauma as a woman who is single and pregnant, we can empathize with her feelings of isolation, alienation, and desperation because of our own experiences. We have seen God comfort and provide in our own situations. We have also seen how God can bring relief and help to people in other situations, such as crisis pregnancies. It's this sense of hopefulness, through God's grace, that I want convey to you, the readers—you, who desire to minister to others who are in crisis, conveying hope to them.

The *Crisis Pregnancy Training Manual*, published by the Christian Action Council, provides a concise definition of *crisis pregnancy*. It is any pregnancy that leads to stress. Under the best circumstances, pregnancy brings major changes to a woman's physical and emotional condition. A married woman can have a crisis pregnancy, even if her child is wanted, when factors such as poverty, illness, and her relationship with her husband lead to stress.

In the majority of cases, however, crisis pregnancy involves single women—very often adolescents—whose pregnancies are not planned. Such women are particularly vulnerable to the upheavals of pregnancy. They often feel completely alone and unable to reach out for help from family and friends. Pregnancy then becomes a catastrophic event that threatens the mother's well-being. It also threatens the emotional well-being of her family and, often, that of her sexual partner. The infant's needs, which cannot be articulated, may not be met, either.

Typically, these women feel that people and circumstances in life are hostile toward them. Even though they may not want to end the child's life, abortion may appear to be the only alternative.

As Christians, we want to be prepared to reach out to these women at this crucial time in their lives. We don't want to condemn them. We must be able to serve them in ways that will meet their special needs.

In preparing this book, I've talked to many women. Their names and certain details have been altered to safeguard confidentiality, but the situations related to them are true. Talking to them gave me a new perspective. It challenged many half-formed notions I had unconsciously developed over the years. As a Christian, I need to view crisis pregnancy with a practical, yet compassionate eye.

Consider:

• *Pregnancy is not a sin.* It's the natural, biological consequence of human sexual activity. Our bodies were created with this function.

• *Sex per se is not a sin.* In its proper context, sexual intercourse is a vital part of a married person's life. A loving Creator designed us with the capacity to enjoy sex. Problems can develop, though, when the timing and participants in some sexual activities are not right. The Bible makes it clear that sexual relations are exclusively intended for heterosexual marriage. Biblical values also reject any abusive or manipulative use of this powerful drive.

• *Sex outside of marriage is a sin, but it is no worse in God's eyes than other sins.* Yet, extramarital sex is worse, humanly speaking, than many other sins because it directly affects other people. Also, sex outside of marriage can have lifetime ramifications. Since extramarital sex can have consequences that are highly visible—a pregnancy—scandal, gossip, and rejection may often follow. A poignant example of Christians who rejected the sinner along with the transgression can be found in Nathaniel Hawthorne's *The Scarlet Letter*. Yet there's very little indication in Scripture of a hierarchy of sins. Jesus makes this point when He equally condemns the sin of lust and the sin of adultery, the sin of anger and the sin of murder. Few of us are aware of people who cheat on their income tax, but God's judgment applies to this "secret" sin just as much as to an all-too-obvious, out-of-wedlock pregnancy.

The essence of the Christian faith is forgiveness and restoration. I view the Church as a hospital. It's there for all people who recognize they have a problem or a need. Each of us has fallen from God's grace through our own sin. In a sense, it's academic whether I become pregnant outside of marriage or steal from my company or hate my boss. The point is, by accepting the forgiveness Christ offers us through His death on the cross, when we repent of our sin, each of us can have a fresh start.

The role of the church is to uphold a consistent standard of love, encourage *everyone* to repent and confess, and receive the reconciliation to God that comes through personal faith in Jesus Christ. But the church must also have a role in the prevention of teen pregnancy and in helping the victims of this crisis.

I am assuming that you are reading this book because you have become aware of or involved with a teen pregnancy situation. I have tried to develop each chapter with you in mind. You, as a concerned Christian, are someone who desires to help people in need, and I pray that this book will be a resource to help you meet those needs.

In preparing this book, Lea has served as technical advisor and liaison to her colleagues and the excellent resources at our local Crisis Pregnancy Center. My role, and that of Dave Jackson, has been to interpret the information and work with the editors at David C. Cook Publishing Co. to arrange it in a practical format you can use. I've depended greatly upon the advice, prayers, and friendship of Lea's colleagues, and I've benefited from contacting other professionals around the country. Let me emphasize, though, that the conclusions are Dave Jackson's and mine. They do not necessarily reflect the opinions of a local Crisis Pregnancy Center or any other organization.

Matt Dacy

CHAPTER ONE

TEEN PREGNANCY — THE SCOPE OF THE PROBLEM

*L*AURA WAS 16 WHEN SHE GOT PREGNANT. *SHE WAS A GOOD student and attended church regularly in the small city where she grew up. She had a real problem with self-worth. Her parents divorced when she was young. Her mother repeatedly stated how worthless Laura's father was, so Laura began to think that she also must be no good since she was his daughter. As a teenager, Laura was looking for a sense of hope and direction, a sense of being loved. But she was looking in all the wrong places.*

Susan, 15, is the somewhat rebellious but popular daughter of a prominent family. She began dating last year, even though her parents thought it was too soon. Her parents travel frequently, and it seemed easier for them to go along with Susan's wishes and activities than to provoke a confrontation. When they were out of town last fall, Susan had a party at her house for friends. Things got out of hand when strangers bringing alcohol and drugs came along with her friends. Now Susan is pregnant, and she's not sure if the boy she'd been dating or someone who had attended the party is the father of her child. Susan's older brother says he'll give her money for an abortion, but Susan isn't sure what to do yet. She hasn't told her parents.

Kathy, 17, lives on her own in a public-housing apartment. She is divorced and has a two-year-old son. Now she is pregnant again. Kathy loves her son, but there is no way she can handle another child. She is determined to get an abortion.

Wanda, 22, dropped out of high school and has had a series of fairly good jobs although she never stays long at any of them. She also has had a series of boyfriends. The last one lived with her for eight or nine months before they broke up. Wanda came to a Crisis Pregnancy Center for help recently when she

9

thought she was pregnant. She learned that wasn't the case and is relieved. Now she says she wants to get her act together. She's not really asking for advice, but it seems like she wants to talk.

Kim, 16, became a Christian four years ago, having grown up in the church. Now has drifted from her faith. Last week she learned she was pregnant. She and her boyfriend want to get married, but her parents refuse to permit it. The boy is not a Christian. Kim is bitter toward God and has walked out on her parents.

Each of the above situations is different. The needs of the girls are different, as are their backgrounds and the support available to them. How would you respond if one of these young women came to you for help? Would you be able to answer her questions? Help her handle her anger? Find resources to meet some of her needs? The intent of this book is to help prepare you to handle situations such as these.

Teen pregnancy—these two words probably conjure up a lot of stereotypical mental pictures. But there is no such thing as a typical pregnant teen. As Christians who desire to help people, we must be aware that the problem of teen pregnancy affects families everywhere—families that are prominent in our churches, low-income families, families of the leaders of our communities, single-parent families, families that go to church only on special occasions. In order to be of help, we need to be as informed as possible.

Teen pregnancy is a serious problem—one that potentially threatens the health and future of the United States. A recent Harris Poll shows that 84 percent of adults in the United States consider teenage pregnancy a major problem. Economics reinforce the point. The Center for Population Options estimates that teen pregnancies annually cost more than $16 billion.

Who is responsible for monitoring this situation? How should society cope with the problem? Could popular media be contributing to it? (A year of typical television programming brings countless scenes of suggested sexual activity into the home, with little attention paid to the consequences of this visual input.)

Much has been written recently in popular and professional

periodicals about the problem of teen pregnancy. According to the National Center for Health Statistics, all measures that describe the incidence of childbearing by unmarried women rose between 1983 and 1984 to the highest levels observed since 1940. These findings indicated that more than one out of every five births in 1984 was to an unmarried mother.

According to an April 29, 1985, issue of *News*, published by the American Medical Association, American teenagers become pregnant more often, have more babies, and have more abortions than teens in any other industrialized nation in the world. Those rates are significantly higher than those of comparable developed countries, the United States being the only one of those countries in which teenage pregnancy has increased in recent years.

Psychology Today has reported that annually one out of ten teenage girls in the United States becomes pregnant, and almost half of these pregnancies result in births—30,000 of them to girls under the age of 15. [1]

Each year, more than a million American teenagers will become pregnant, according to *Time* magazine. Four out of five of them are unmarried. [2] If present trends continue, researchers estimate, fully 40 percent of today's 14-year-old girls will be pregnant at least once before the age of 20.

Who Is Getting Pregnant and Why?

The problem is not limited to certain geographical regions or specific age groups or income strata. In fact, it is increasing with remarkable speed among socioeconomic groups that have long dismissed teen pregnancy as something that happens to "other" people. Today, white, middle-class families, Christians among them, are experiencing teen pregnancy in record numbers.

Since many teens lack the maturity to make long-term plans and have poor academic skills, pregnancy often becomes the result of choices made by these young people. Strange as it may seem, many teens—male and female—want to have a baby. *Psychology Today* lists several reasons for this:

1. A baby is someone to love in a harsh environment.
2. Pregnancy brings attention.
3. Pregnancy is a way to trap a reluctant partner into a longer-term relationship.

11

4. Pregnancy is a way to assert independence—for a boy to prove his manhood and a girl to become her mother's equal.

5. Having children is a method to "keep up" with friends who are having them.

6. There is nothing else to do; to begin a family seems like an interesting, temporary activity. [3]

Changing Patterns of Sexuality

Is anything different about teenagers today? There have always been students who have done poorly in school. Insecurity and self-doubt are not new issues with which teens struggle. And if you look at numbers alone, the rate of teen pregnancy was higher in 1957 than it is today. But that year was in an era of early marriages: 25 percent of all Americans aged 18-20 were married. The vast majority of teen births occurred to girls who were 17 or older, but they were married. During these years, high school was the time to work through the problems of becoming mature. Students who did not excel academically had the opportunity to prepare for a viable vocational career. Things have changed considerably in the past 30 years.

What is different today is that more teens are sexually active outside of marriage and at younger ages than ever before. It has become a common expression to say that the sexual revolution has moved from college campuses to high schools—and now to junior highs. *Time* magazine, in the December 9, 1985, issue, quoted a Johns Hopkins study that reveals one out of five 15-year-olds has had sex; so have 33 percent of 16-year-olds and 43 percent of those 17 years old.

Psychology Today reported: "Today, among 15- to 17-year-olds in this country, almost half of the boys and a third of the girls are sexually active." [4] In fact, the rate of increase in sexual activity is highest among white adolescent girls. The rate of pregnancy for white American teens is higher than the pregnancy rate in most developed countries. *Time* recorded these statistics: in 1950, fewer than 15 percent of teen births were out of wedlock; today they are more than 50 percent; and in some communities they range up to 75 percent. [5]

Contraceptive Confusion

American teens are sexually sophisticated as never before, but a key characteristic of adolescence remains unchanged—many teens are woefully ignorant about the facts of reproduction. For over a decade schools have provided intensive sex education, but folk myths and peer misperceptions do not die quickly or easily. Myths, such as "you can't get pregnant the first time" and "you can't get pregnant if you make love standing up" can still be heard. Teens who are sexually active are usually reluctant to use contraception. They tend to believe they are too young to become pregnant, and they presume they are safe because they have intercourse infrequently or at the wrong time of the month. Rarely does a teen use a contraceptive for the first sexual encounter. Many sexually active teens feel that using precautions removes the romance and spontaneity, the feeling of "getting carried away." Having to prepare for intercourse makes it seem planned and contrived, and consequently, less forgivable.

It seems apparent that, in spite of sexual sophistication, when it comes to dealing with their own sexuality, teens are in over their heads. They need both accurate information and help in forming values to guide them in making responsible choices that will serve the best interests of those involved.

Post-teen Unwed Pregnancy

While in her 20s, Laura, described earlier in this chapter, became pregnant again. This pregnancy was a deliberate choice made at the suggestion of her current boyfriend with the hope of strengthening their weak relationship. That tactic did not work. Laura found herself a single parent with two daughters by different fathers.

Although the focus of this book will be on pregnant teenagers, another segment of our population increasingly suffers the problem of crisis pregnancy. This segment involves women who have passed their teen years. Increasing numbers of women are postponing marriage or becoming divorced and, by being sexually active, are at risk of unplanned pregnancies. The problems that these women have during a crisis pregnancy may not seem as "dramatic" as those of a tenth grader, but the difficulties are no less real. And the individual lives of mother and child are no less important.

The National Center for Health Statistics confirms that women past age 20 accounted for 59 percent of all unwed births in 1980. In 1984, their share of these births rose to 65 percent. Women past age 20 are beginning to edge out teenagers as the ones most likely to give birth out of wedlock. Future years should show an ever-increasing disparity among these groups.

A Self-perpetuating Problem

Perhaps the most cruel irony of crisis pregnancy is that so few people seem to learn from experience. *Time* magazine noted that 82 percent of the girls who gave birth at age 15 or younger were themselves daughters of teenage mothers. It's an alarming thought to realize that in as short a time as every 12 years this cycle can repeat itself. [6] Some of these young mothers will become grandmothers in their 20s.

Teen mothers have more children more frequently than other mothers. Less than two years separate the births of first and second children for 57 percent of mothers ages 18 to 19. This was true for only 32 percent of mothers ages 20-24 and 14 percent of those aged 30-34 years. In fact, about 15 percent of this year's pregnant teens will become pregnant again in a year; and 30 percent of them will be expecting in two more years.

Author Marian Wright Edelman has concluded that teen pregnancy is inversely related to positive self-esteem.[7] In other words, the more negative self-esteem that a girl has, the more likely she is to become pregnant. Girls with low self-esteem seem to be missing a sense of hope for the future. According to Virginia Satir, family therapist and author of *Peoplemaking,* self-esteem is learned at home and tends to be cyclical—parents with positive self-esteem tend to rear children with positive self-esteem. [8] Thus, the problem of poor self-esteem, which Edelman identified as correlating with a high teen pregnancy rate, can be self-perpetuating.

The Global Perspective

The dimensions of this problem become clearer when you look at the situation from a global perspective. The Guttmacher Institute did just that and concluded that teen birth rates in the United States are higher by a wide margin than those of other developed nations.

The contrast is especially vivid for younger teens. The United States has more than five births per 1,000 girls who are 14 years old. This rate is almost four times that of Canada, the only other country with even one birth per 1,000 girls that age. Overall, the pregnancy rate for American girls ages 15-19 is 96 per 1,000. This compares with 14 per 1,000 in the Netherlands, 35 in Sweden, 43 in France, 44 in Canada, and 45 in England.

Teen Pregnancy and the Black Community

Unwed pregnancy is a serious threat to the black community. Statistics show the pregnancy rate for unwed black teens is considerably higher than that for whites, but the gap between the two groups is narrowing as the pregnancy rate for white teens is increasing rapidly.

Here are some statistics:

• A study by the Guttmacher Institute found that almost half of all black females in the United States are pregnant by age 20. Nearly 90 percent of those babies are reared in fatherless homes.

• In 1982, 56.5 percent of all black children were born to unwed mothers. [9] Contrast the above rate with about 33 percent of black infants in 1965.

Black leadership groups, such as the National Urban League, have targeted teenage pregnancy as a major concern for the black community. Urban League leaders cite teenage pregnancy as a leading force in unemployment, dropout rates in school, and the number of blacks living below the poverty line. These organizations, as well as churches within the communities, are actively addressing the need for education and reform in this area.

• Teen pregnancy is less of a problem among other ethnic groups according to the NCHS. Childbearing is relatively uncommon among Chinese, Japanese, Filipino, and other Asian and Pacific Island teens. In 1984, these groups had six percent of their total births to women younger than age 20. (Eleven percent of all white births were to teen mothers, as were 20 percent of Native American and Latin births and 16 percent of Hawaiian births.)

What Are the Choices?

At age 15, Mary Anne became the only Christian in her home, but she didn't have encouragement to get involved with a church or youth group. In her large family, no one paid much attention to her. At her part-time job she met a young man who did. Soon she was pregnant. Getting no support from home, she saw a newspaper ad for a Christian home for unwed mothers. There she received counsel about the choices available to her.

Adoption was not an easy choice, but she knew it was right for her. She says she still has hard, sad times—like Mother's Day—knowing that her son is growing up without knowing she is his mother. But she is confident that this was the best choice for him in spite of how hard it is for her.

When a teenager finds out she is pregnant, life-changing choices must be considered. Confusion, fear, and uncertainty usually accompany this news. Time seems of the essence, and pressure can mount from a host of sources—boyfriend, parents, friends, counselors. Many of these people may disagree among themselves, which can leave the pregnant teen feeling as if she's in a vacuum.

There are basically four options for the teen to consider, but not all of them are acceptable to every teen:

• Parent alone—by far the most popular option among some socioeconomic and ethnic groups;

• Marriage—a choice which all too often ends in divorce unless the parents of the couple are fully supportive of the marriage and are actively, positively involved in the lives of the expectant parents;

• Adoption—a desirable choice, especially for younger teens;

• Abortion—the preferred choice by many teens, but especially for many Christians, it is not an option.

How do today's teens respond to these choices? Here are a few statistics that show some of the results of their decisions:

• Fewer than 5 percent of teen mothers place their babies for adoption (as opposed to about 35 percent in the early 1960s).

• About 45 percent of pregnant teens have abortions. That is why the birth rate is declining even though the rate of teen pregnancy continues to increase. Nearly 30 percent of all abortions in the United States are performed on teenagers. Most of these young mothers are from middle and upper economic classes. The Guttmacher Institute has documented that by age 18, 60 out of every 1,000 American girls has had an abortion. This compares to about 7 girls per 1,000 in the Netherlands, 24 per 1,000 in Canada, and 20 per 1,000 in England and Wales. That makes the U.S. abortion rate higher than the *combined* totals of these other leading industrial countries.

At 16, Diane got pregnant the first time she had intercourse.

She had just started dating a few months earlier. Diane and her parents, who were regular church attenders, did not consult anyone for advice concerning this crisis pregnancy. They decided abortion was the best solution for Diane—the suggestion made by their family physician.

Curt Young, executive director of the Christian Action Council, notes that overall "at least ten percent of women of childbearing age have had one abortion."[10] The Center for Disease Control estimates the number of abortions in America to have increased at least tenfold from the days before legalization of abortion to the present.

Increasing numbers of pregnant teens who reject abortion as an option choose to keep their babies and parent alone, especially those in lower socioeconomic groups. Usually these young mothers require welfare assistance. Childbirth "forces" these girls into instant adulthood, bypassing the more normal psychosocial developmental process.

Fathers: The Forgotten Factor

Tim was the 16-year-old son of key leaders in a large church. He had just started dating Evelyn, who was 15. Her family attended the church but was not active in it. When Evelyn became pregnant, Tim's family tried to dominate the situation. He was kept out of discussions and forbidden to date her. After the baby was born and Evelyn decided to keep her, Tim's parents changed their attitudes about the situation. They helped Tim work out ways to pay for child care. He had a part-time job during high school. While in college, his parents took over the child support on a loan basis. Tim will repay them after graduation. He plans to continue supporting his daughter even though he has no plans to marry Evelyn.

It seems that researchers are just now discovering what most teens learn in a hurry—that it takes two people to make a baby. In the past, intensive studies have documented all aspects of pregnancy as they relate to mother and child, but the fathers have received scant attention. They are, of course, part of the problem. They also suffer its consequences and must play a role in any meaningful solution.

Clearly, many of these adolescent males share the immaturity that can mark teen mothers. Teen fathers, in spite of the fact that early sexual encounters are usually unsatisfactory, are often happy about impregnating their girlfriends because they think it affirms their arrival into manhood.

But it's unfair to dismiss these boys as hit-and-run artists. As researchers probe the feelings of teen fathers, they discover a far more complex picture. Many have a strong desire to "do right" by the mother. Today, this may not mean marriage, but it may mean providing for the mother and child financially. Because they usually come from broken homes themselves, these boys have little understanding of what a father's role should include.

In general, teen fathers have less education, lower incomes, and more offspring than men who postpone siring children until their twenties. Unfortunately, the most committed teen father often aggravates his initial problem of creating a pregnancy by quitting school. At best, his hope of getting a job is a very short-term solution that restricts future chances for the new family's stability and prosperity.

At the same time, professional guidance proves remarkably successful in helping teen fathers. *Time* magazine quoted a promising study that examined counseling, job-skill services, and parenting classes which were offered to about 400 teenage fathers in eight cities.[11] The two-year program found that 82 percent of the men had daily contact with their children, 74 percent assisted with the child's financial support, and 90 percent kept up a relationship with the mother. Of special note is that 46 percent of the men who had dropped out of school resumed their education, while 61 percent of previously unemployed fathers landed jobs.

At the other end of the spectrum, when women choose to have an abortion, the fathers often are left out of the decision-making process. Current laws in most places state that men do not have the right to decide or even know whether the mothers of their children have had abortions.

Yet, these fathers often share the emotional trauma. Arthur Shostak, a sociologist at Drexal University, wrote *Men and Abortion: Lessons, Losses and Love.* He believes that abortion is a vast, unrecognized source of tension for men—which many of them endure without support. The men he interviewed felt guilty, bitter, and, most of all, helpless. While many of these men opposed a law that would prohibit abortion, their eagerness to share responsibility for the decisions of pregnancy raises troubling questions for those who insist abortion is a woman's private, exclusive right.

Time magazine noted that Planned Parenthood refused to allow Shostak to distribute his survey at centers that perform abortions. *Time* commented, "That hard-line view may owe something to the fear that attention to males at clinics will ultimately raise moral qualms about abortion . . . . Shostak thinks the matter is simple: it takes two to make a pregnancy, and like it or not, both are involved in the result."[12]

For people who want to help alleviate the problem of teen pregnancy, it is just and practical to serve the needs of men as well as of women and children.

Profile of a Pregnant Teen

Although each person is unique and in unique circumstances, common threads can be found that frequently characterize teen pregnancy situations. This composite was adapted from one developed by the House of His Creation in Coatesville, Pennsylvania.

Her Background

She is likely to come from a single-parent home. This fact is significant in two ways: (a) she may have a negative father image; (b) most of the time, she has only had her mother as a role model for parenting and communicating skills. If her home is intact, both parents are likely to work outside the home.

Her Feelings

She has a deep, inner sense of joy that comes from the knowledge that she is nurturing a new life. This feeling of joy is centered on the baby, but this joy can be countered by negative emotions from diverse sources. She may have a sense of personal worthlessness from a poor self-image, which is intensified by her personal crisis. She is confused by all the decisions that she must make; she may change her mind frequently and often act impulsively. She is probably experiencing anger—anger at herself, the father of her unborn child, and her parents. As a young person, she may be angry at being thrust into a world of adult-like decision making so quickly. She also is probably feeling guilty because of her sexual activity.

Her Pressures

Her life is full of pressures from various sources during this crisis. Pressures from people—parents, sexual partners, friends, and others who may give conflicting advice; pressures from circumstances, like finances, living situations, physical condition, work, and school; pressures from society because of its emphasis on sex without guilt and abortion on demand.

Her Potential

She has a desire to nurture life, but it is difficult for her to find support for this task. She also has a value system and beliefs. Even if these may not be fully thought out, they need to be respected but challenged, if necessary, in a caring, supportive environment. She has dreams and hopes for her life, but she needs someone who believes in her, someone who will help her attain her goals.

This young mother-to-be has been created in the image of God. She is a unique and special individual, but she may need help to fully realize this.

Impact of Pregnancy on the Teenage Girl

Teen pregnancy affects all members of a family but most of all the expectant mother. Consequences range from economic concerns to matters of health. Problems can begin almost immediately and sometimes extend through the lifetimes of the people involved.

• Pregnancy itself is a risk to young teens. Their bodies lack the physical maturity to endure the stresses of pregnancy and nourish the baby as successfully as women in their twenties. Girls younger than age 15 face a higher death rate from complications. Malnutrition and premature and prolonged labor are special problems for teens.

• Two out of three pregnant teenagers drop out of school, according to March of Dimes. Some teen mothers eventually finish high school, but that total number is less than 50 percent of all women who gave birth before age 18. By contrast, 96 percent of women who postpone childbirth until their twenties do complete high school.

• Limited education for mothers translates into restricted opportunities in the work force. This only compounds the problems of having another mouth to feed, the need for child care, and the probable absence of a father's emotional and financial support.

• Income potential for a teenage mother is half of what her peers can expect. Dependency upon family members and/or welfare is likely.

• Barely one-third of pregnant teens marry the fathers of their children, reported the Guttmacher Institute. Unfortunately, those who do marry face harsh odds. Americans who marry during their teens are two to three times more apt to divorce than people who delay marriage until their twenties.

Impact on the Infant

Teen pregnancy poses special difficulties for the person least able to correct the situation—the baby.

Problems may start well before delivery. The American College of Obstetricians and Gynecologists recommends that a pregnant woman make about 13 visits for prenatal medical care during the course of a normal full-term pregnancy. Teen mothers tend to begin prenatal care later and make fewer total visits than do other women. For example, in 1984, according to the National Center for Health Statistics, 21 percent of mothers at greatest risk (those younger than 15 years of age, regardless of race) had inadequate prenatal care. In addition, teen mothers often add dangerous life-style habits to their lack of proper medical care. Junk food, alcohol consumption, late hours, and drugs are harmful to both mother and child.

Sexual Activity among Churched Teens

Even though her home life had been very difficult, Constance became a strong, active Christian during high school. Partly to escape problems at home, she went away to Bible college. She was particularly drawn to missions. She reflected later that this was probably an attempt to escape even further. While working for a short time in an Asian refugee camp, she became pregnant by a national government worker. Her need to be loved and accepted followed her halfway around the world.

Little encouragement can be found to indicate that teens within our churches are less sexually involved than teens outside the church. Search Institute of Minneapolis, Minnesota, conducted a study in 1984 of 10,000 *churched* adolescents. Their findings revealed that over 20 percent of junior-high-age boys (seventh through ninth grade) had engaged in sexual intercourse. The statistic for girls was 10 percent. (Other studies have shown that once sexual activity begins, it is likely to continue.)

21

In 1981 a Gallup youth survey indicated that 52 percent of churchgoing teens felt that premarital sex was not wrong. Though this is considerably lower than the 77 percent rate of nonattenders, it reveals an alarming disregard for Scripture's teaching of abstinence outside of marriage.

Churched teens appear to conform to peer and cultural pressures in areas of sexual behavior. It's as if they're hearing two messages: one from parents, the church, and Christian schooling which says "no" to sexual activity outside of marriage; and the other from peers, the media, and contemporary secular society which says, "Go ahead. Enjoy sex! You have the right."

Christian teens today do not "stumble" into sexual intercourse out of ignorance. They are aware of sexual behavior and its consequences. Yet, many who are sexually active will state that they rarely use birth control because it would indicate they were planning to sin. Many prefer not to make that conscious decision even though they subconsciously realize that societal pressures make it hard to resist sexual involvement. Should they become pregnant, most of these girls expect to marry the fathers of their babies.

Somehow those of us who are leaders and teachers in our churches and who have a special concern for teens must help them realize the connection between the absolutes taught in Scripture and their own conduct.

These are just some of the facts that provide a grim overview of the problem of teen pregnancy. Each one of the statistics represents a person. In the next chapter are stories of young women—members of families in our congregations, daughters of our neighbors, even members of our own families—which can help us learn how to best reach out, support, and help them in this crisis.

CHAPTER TWO

CASE STUDIES

THERE ARE NO *TYPICAL* CASE STUDIES OF TEEN PREGNANCY. Each case is unique and must be addressed with sensitivity, compassion, and understanding. Here are some important variables that can affect every situation: quality of the relationship with the father of the baby; support of the parents; economic situation; ethnic background; age of the teen; and ability to take responsibility. This chapter contains a representation of situations involving teen pregnancy. The stories are presented with details changed to allow individuals to remain anonymous. They are to help you understand the emotions, problems, and implications of teenage pregnancies.

Amy—A Case for Adoption

Amy enjoyed life and lots of friends. She was a delightful, carefree 16-year-old. Carefree, that is, until her pregnancy, when the consequences of sexual activity became obvious. Then the happy-go-lucky attitude was exchanged for one that reflected the weight of the decision she soon had to make about the baby.

Amy's parents married at age 19, soon after her mother became pregnant. They divorced several years later. Amy lives with her mother but sees her father regularly. All members of her family are Christians, though the pressures of the parents' work have kept them from being very involved in their respective churches.

Amy's pregnancy was especially surprising to her mother because she thought she had an open relationship with Amy. She felt that Amy was confiding honestly her dating life. They enjoyed each other as good friends. To Amy's father, her pregnancy was a painful shock because it seemed that his sin was being passed on to his children.

Amy had been dating Brad for several months, but he broke up with her after learning she was pregnant. Right from the start, Amy wanted to keep her baby. She kept talking about how excited she was, how much fun it would be, how she'd enjoy having a baby to love.

Her parents, though no longer married to each other, supported Amy during this crisis. They sensed that Amy was not thinking objectively about her ability to parent nor about what would be best for the child. They sought advice from several sources— pastoral, school, and family counselors. They attended sessions with Amy and also encouraged her to be counseled individually.

Finally, through self-evaluation and the prayers and support of clergy, counselors, and family, Amy decided that adoption was best for everyone involved. This would assure that her baby would be reared in a home with two mature, Christian parents who could provide for the baby what Amy could not.

This decision was difficult and painful. Regardless of her age, a mother never forgets a child she has carried. But Amy has come to celebrate her choice. She sacrificed her own desires to choose what would be best for her child.

Christine—Setting New Directions

Christine was reared in a Christian home and accepted Jesus Christ as her Savior at age 11. She generally got along well with her parents.

During the summer after her junior year in high school, Christine began to date Scott. He was two years older than she and was studying at the local vocational school.

Scott was Christine's first serious boyfriend. He had grown up in a nominally Christian home but never made a personal commitment of faith. He'd been sexually involved with two previous girlfriends, but the relationships meant little to him. Christine was special. After their third or fourth date, he began to ask her for sex.

"He didn't pressure me or manipulate me," she says. "Since we talked about getting married sometime, that made me think it was okay."

Christine and her mother had discussed sexual matters during a couple of awkward conversations a few years earlier. At the time, Christine was confused by the subject and not really interested. Her mother seemed relieved to let the matter drop. Neither of them had brought it up again.

Christine knew her parents would never buy contraceptives for her, and she was afraid she'd be in trouble if she purchased birth control devices and her mother found them at home. Consequently, Christine took no precautions.

This began a double life for Christine. She continued to participate in church activities, even bringing Scott along. At the same time, she was sexually active and rather pleased to have such an exciting "secret world." Less than six months into the relationship, though, she became pregnant. Her secret world fell apart. "I was scared to tell my folks—but, most of all, I felt I let them down," she says now.

Christine's parents were stunned. Her father says, "Christine was a good girl; she never gave us any trouble. I thought we were doing the right thing by not inserting ourselves into her life." Today, he realizes that what he thought was the "right thing" was really a tolerance of a superficial relationship with his daughter.

Despite the stress of this crisis, the family rallied. Christine and her mother saw a Christian counselor. Christine's faith deepened as she grasped the seriousness of her problem and saw the forgiveness and help available to her.

Though Christianity was still irrelevant to Scott, he promised to abstain from any further sexual involvement with Christine. He volunteered to drive her to a special school for teen mothers and supported her decision to place their baby for adoption.

But four months into her pregnancy, Christine miscarried. This was as shocking to her parents as had been the news that she was pregnant.

"We had covered this situation in prayer," her mother said. "We were committed to doing what was right for all parties concerned—including the baby. Then everything was swept from our hands." For Christine's parents, this was a crisis in faith. It took several weeks for them to accept their helplessness. They had to stand back and trust God, knowing that He is supreme and in control.

Christine adjusted to this loss more easily since, from the day of the miscarriage, she believed her infant was safe in the Lord's care. She had been planning to place the child for adoption with a Christian family. "We were determined to see good come out of the situation."

Now Christine is using this experience to allow the Lord to purify her lifestyle. She says she wants to use her energy to live as a godly person.

"I can't return to being a virgin," she says, "but I've recommitted all the details of my life to God. That gives me a fresh start."

Laura—A Struggling Single Parent

(Laura, referred to in Chapter One, has two children by different fathers. She came from a strife-filled home, had church upbringing, and was a good student. As Laura explains, she was looking for a sense of hope and direction for her life—most of all, a sense of being loved, not for what she did, but for who she was.)

I was 16 the first time I got pregnant.

I realize now that I had a real problem with self-worth. Every bad thing that happened to me just made it worse. My parents fought a lot. My mom said over and over that my dad was a no-good, and I got to thinking, "He's part of me. I must be bad, too."

My big desire was to be loved. I never heard of being loved just for who you are. I thought you had to give in to other people and then maybe they'd love you. I'm sure the guys I knew could sense this, and they exploited it. So the times when I agreed to have sex, I felt used.

In school, we'd covered the facts of life from fifth grade on, including high-school health class. But I didn't connect that information to what I was doing personally.

Part of the problem was a lack of support at home. I remember coming home, excited about what I was learning, and Mom making it perfectly clear that in no way did she want to talk about it. That left me pretty much on my own.

At school, you'd talk about sex with your friends. Everyone knew who was sleeping together, and on Monday the big question was, "How far did you get?"

But there sure was a double standard. I was one of the first in my class to get pregnant. It was during my sophomore year. There was a big scandal, lots of whispers. When I got pregnant, I felt cut off from my friends. Most of my family was indifferent—"You got yourself into this." Either people turned on me or they left me alone.

I knew what contraceptives were and pretty much how to use them. There were posters in school and a clinic where you could get them. It was a status thing for girls to go together to the clinic. A friend knew I was getting serious about this guy, so she'd invited me to go—like an initiation.

I had used birth control, but then I went off of it. Maybe it didn't seem natural, or I couldn't relate it with what could happen nine months later.

In my school, it was understood that it was up to the girl to take precautions. The guys were too macho—no way would they do that. The girls basically thought, "Somebody's got to think of this," so they went along and acted like it was sophisticated.

I can tell you how that attitude makes a girl suffer in the long run, because if you get pregnant, everyone acts like it's all your fault. "She's some kind of tramp," or "She's a fool," or "She's just trying to trap him." That's what they said. Sometimes girls said it about each other.

I turned 17 during my first pregnancy. I was still a minor and very much under everyone's influence. According to them, I didn't have much of what you'd call a real choice. In my family and my neighborhood, you got married. That was it. Everyone pushed, but I wouldn't give in. I had no love for the guy. That's one thing I'm proud of—that I wouldn't knuckle into that pressure. But being a single mom was rough. I felt ignored and put down. I pretty much dropped out of church.

My second child was planned. I wasn't married then, either. The guy and I had been going together for a couple of years. We'd live together, then break up. He asked me to get pregnant, and I thought a child would bring us closer together. That's what I always heard children are supposed to do. So in this case I deliberately chose to avoid using birth control. Even if they were giving it away on the street corner, you couldn't have talked me into using it. What I really needed at the time was a sense of value and personal direction. I was 21 then, and living on my own. It was my boyfriend's idea, and I thought it would strengthen our relationship.

That's not how it worked out, and within a few months, he was pressing me to get an abortion. "Just get rid of it," he'd say, like a baby was something you could take a pass on if you weren't interested anymore. That's when I began to say, "Hold it."

I decided to keep the baby, even though I knew our relationship was over. Now I'm a single mother with two daughters by different fathers. It's hard sometimes. A lot of people ask why I didn't place my kids for adoption. I don't want to speak for anyone else, but in my case, that just wouldn't be right.

My daughters have different fathers, but I was attracted to them for basically the same reasons. They were good-looking, a little older, and higher up on the social scale. One of them had plenty of money. Both times, the guys' families took the pregnancy as a big scandal. I really felt put down. One of the guys even questioned whether it was his child I was carrying.

I'm sorry to say that both guys sensed my weakness—I was hurting to be loved. Both wound up being physically abusive to me. The first guy took out his frustrations by hitting me. The second one laid a hand on me within the first month we were going out. But I still stuck with him, thinking I could change him. Maybe I was afraid to be alone.

I became a Christian after the second guy left me. Now I see that I was worshiping these men and not the Lord. I wanted so much to give love and be loved, but these guys were not the answer. They had their own problems, and besides, no human can give you the complete acceptance that Jesus can.

Laura has worked hard to maintain a good relationship with the fathers of her children so that the girls will be comfortably involved with them. As her daughters get older, they're able to see needs that their fathers have. They are praying that these men will come to know the Lord.

Laura found help at a local Crisis Pregnancy Center during her second pregnancy. She found acceptance from the staff and, during that time, dedicated her life to Christ.

She senses the blessing of God on her young single-parent family even though parenting alone is difficult. She's found a good church that she attends with her mother. Much of the pain of the past is being erased. Even in the rough times, she senses God's peace. Most of all, she has never regretted her decisions to keep her daughters.

With the child support provided by the fathers and part-time employment, Laura is able to care for her family. She also volunteers her time in several ways—at an alcohol treatment center, in a ministry to blind people, and in the singles group at her church.

Laura knows that her daughters will have many questions as they grow up. She plans to answer them as best she can but also point the girls to someone to whom they can turn, no matter what—they can turn to God. Laura summarizes her circumstances in this way: "Today, the girls and I are a family, and with the Lord's help, we're making it."

Dawn—An Abortion Changed Her Life

"At the time, there seemed to be no alternative. It was rush, rush, hurry up."

Dawn is now 25 years old. Seven years ago, when she was a senior in high school and had just been awarded a scholarship to a prestigious college, she found out she was pregnant.

It was a crisis in Dawn's family, but none of the family members sought advice or counsel. "We all wanted a quick solution," she recalls. "I think we were all ashamed." Dawn had been counting on an enjoyable senior year of high school, and her parents had great hopes for her college career.

The emotional pressure of the circumstances built. Dawn's boyfriend, Mel, broke up with her when she told him about the pregnancy. He refused to be involved in the situation. Dawn's parents wanted to avoid a scandal, so they didn't press matters with him. Nobody liked the idea of an abortion, but it seemed the best way to get on with normal family life.

Dawn's parents say they are Christians and attend church, but it is not a central part of their lives. They see little relationship between the teachings of the Bible and issues such as the sanctity of life.

The abortion took place in the spring of Dawn's senior year. Her parents made sure she was well cared for medically. Dawn recalls, "It wasn't brutal, but I still had this feeling like I was an object on an assembly line." Afterward, her pregnancy was never spoken of at home.

Dawn went away to a well-known college where she became involved with a fellowship group on campus. There she made a personal commitment to Jesus Christ. She was able to resolve her intense feelings of guilt about the abortion, but a sense of regret remained. "I had killed a child to be sure my own plan worked out," Dawn says, "when all the time God was able to do better than I ever could . . . . But I never asked Him."

Dawn became popular and held leadership positions in her campus group. For more than two years she did not tell friends about her abortion, though she did confide in a faculty member. As this relationship grew and her faith developed, Dawn felt the need to speak out. In time, she became a leader on campus for the pro-life position. Speaking out on these issues became a form of healing, though her parents were unhappy that this family secret was being made public.

Dawn now works as an office administrator and is active in a local church. When the occasion arises, she is willing to talk about her experience. She has been quoted in the newspaper on the subject and by a Christian magazine.

"It's ironic," she says. "I wanted my pregnancy to end quickly and then put it behind me. But the action I took—abortion—has led me into a more public role than I could have imagined. I thought I had no choice, but the Bible makes it clear that we all have choices and we should choose life."

Through this abortion, which Dawn realizes was sin, she has experienced God's forgiveness in a profound way.

Beth—Married, but It's Not Easy

Beth was 19 when she became pregnant. She knew her relationship with Greg had gotten too physical. They had tried double dating, group activities, study parties—anything to avoid sexual intimacy. These measures worked for a while, but they were not adequate. "The crazy thing is, we were bragging to each other how well the `hands-off' policy was working," Beth said. "We had reduced the number of times we had intercourse, and I was being extra careful. Obviously, that was no solution!"

Greg and Beth were attending a small Christian college. That environment made things difficult for them. "At a small school," Beth recalled, "nothing remains secret very long. Some kids were nice about it, but I felt put down by teachers I had trusted and even by some of my friends."

Greg and Beth knew abortion was out of the question, and Beth also had misgivings about adoption. They cared for each other, so they decided to get engaged.

That decision came just as the president of the college hinted that disciplinary action would have to be taken. A single mother would not be allowed on campus, so the only way Beth could remain enrolled was to get married. There was no mention that Greg might face expulsion. Beth became cynical about the double standard. She talked to her pastor and the college chaplain, but kept many of these feelings under cover.

The wedding took place. Greg kept focusing his energy on his job and campus sports activities, taking no spiritual leadership in the marriage. Beth wanted to continue classes, but her parents cut off financial support because they felt she should concentrate on being a mother.

Forced to sacrifice her education because of the pregnancy, Beth became angry. Bitterness entered her relationship with Greg; by their first anniversary, they were barely speaking to each other.

At the encouragement of her parents, Beth and Greg began

marriage counseling. In time, they realized that *doing* the right thing—getting married—was not enough. They had gone through the motions without a strong commitment to each other and without plans and goals for the future. These newlyweds were surprised when happiness did not follow automatically.

Beth began to gain insight into her feelings of anger and bitterness. "I see now that I had never forgiven myself for having sex before marriage," says Beth. "It was something I wanted to do, but it violated the ideas I had held dear for a long time."

Greg says, "We didn't realize that we had to do more than solve a problem pregnancy. We had to build a future for ourselves."

After several months of regular counseling, Beth and Greg began putting a *real* marriage together. They are grateful that they were able to rescue their relationship before it was too late. Greg has promised that soon, when their son is older, Beth will be able to resume her education on a part-time basis.

A Parent's Perspective

"It's very difficult to watch your young daughter 'blossom' into the final stages of pregnancy," Anne said, as she reflected on Elizabeth's unexpected pregnancy. "Being with her through labor was especially hard."

Having had four children, Anne knew well what lay ahead for her 16-year-old daughter. At first Anne felt angry that Elizabeth had allowed herself to get into this situation. But the anger was soon replaced with pity toward her daughter who, in many ways, seemed more like a child than a woman. Anne and her husband were middle-income parents living in a town of 40,000. Elizabeth was the second child, the first daughter. Anne and her husband had grown up in families that didn't talk much about feelings and experiences. It was not surprising that the children, especially Elizabeth, did not talk much about what was going on in their lives. Yet there were loving relationships among family members.

Though Anne has faith in God, she was uncomfortable in church. Her husband and children never attended, so the family was essentially without spiritual support during this crisis.

Elizabeth became pregnant during her junior year of high school. She and her boyfriend had been dating for several months. They felt certain that they were "in love," and they planned to marry right after high school.

As Anne watched her daughter, she began noticing changes in Elizabeth's body. About a month later, Elizabeth told her mother that she was pregnant. (Elizabeth and a friend had gone to a clinic to confirm the condition.)

Since Anne had observed physical changes in Elizabeth that indicated she might be pregnant, Elizabeth's announcement of the fact did not come as a shock to Anne. But it was shocking to the boyfriend, so shocking that he wanted nothing to do with Elizabeth from then on. He even threatened to harm Elizabeth physically if she told his parents. This tense relationship added to the stress of this crisis. Elizabeth's father initially had strong negative feelings about the pregnancy but resolved them and began to assist with decision making.

Anne was embarrassed when relatives had to be told and when the result of Elizabeth's actions became obvious to everyone. She was also embarrassed by what the situation might imply about the family and about her as a mother.

As Elizabeth's senior year approached, Anne spent a lot of time helping her consider options. Elizabeth wanted to finish high school; she took the remaining required courses plus special classes in prenatal and child care. This allowed Elizabeth to maintain contact with many supportive friends and make new friends who were in similar circumstances.

Anne had suggested counseling to help her daughter sort through feelings and options, but Elizabeth refused to consider it. Anne also suggested that adoption might be a good solution, but since Anne felt it was something she herself could not do, that option was presented weakly. Still, Anne felt Elizabeth was too close to the "doll" stage of childhood to think realistically about parenting. As far as Elizabeth was concerned, keeping the baby was the only alternative.

Anne became the grandmother of a baby girl in January, just a few days after her daughter finished her high school requirements. The father of the baby came to see Elizabeth the next day but had no contact with her after that. His parents ask about their grandchild from time to time.

Anne's granddaughter is now four years old. Elizabeth and the child have always lived with Anne. At times this is frustrating for Anne; it's hard not to be actively involved in rearing her granddaughter as long as Elizabeth is living there, even though Anne knows it is primarily Elizabeth's responsibility. Sometimes it's confusing for the child to have two "moms."

In many ways Anne is glad that Elizabeth and the child have lived with her, because Elizabeth has not always been a responsible parent. Yet Anne knows that as long as Elizabeth can rely on her for so much, Elizabeth may possibly never be motivated to become more responsible.

Looking back over the past four years, Anne wishes she could do two things differently: insist that Elizabeth receive counseling, and help Elizabeth live on her own while being supportive and involved in her life.

Many of the expectant mothers in these case studies had no mediator or support person. One can only speculate on how these stories might have been different if a caring, loving Christian had been there to help.

Though the cases you face may vary, God's grace covers *all* situations when people turn to Him in submission and trust. This is the most important message you can bring to unmarried pregnant teens, expectant fathers, and their families.

CHAPTER THREE

QUESTIONS AND ANSWERS

W E ASKED SOCIAL WORKERS, YOUTH PASTORS, COUN-
selors—people who work with pregnant teenagers—
what questions these young people have when they
come for help. The consensus among professionals is that, as in
other crises involving children and youth, those involved rarely
ask questions. Rather, they usually make statements that must be
sensitively probed.

This chapter presents some of the common issues that pregnant teens bring up and suggests ways of handling them. In addition to concerns of the expectant teen parents, likely questions
from the grandparents and people in the church also are included. These questions and answers provide *general* guidelines.
This information will need to be adapted to your situation and
the needs of the person you are helping.

Concerns of Pregnant Teens

I can't believe I'm pregnant! We had sex only a couple of times.

It's possible to get pregnant the first and maybe only time you
have intercourse. *Anytime* contact between the sex organs of a
fertile male and a fertile female occurs, pregnancy is a possibility. (Note: Since pregnancy can happen to very young teens, it
may be appropriate for the helper to include an explanation of
how pregnancy occurs.)

*My boyfriend said I couldn't get pregnant if we made love
standing up.*

There's an endless list of folk notions about avoiding pregnancy. Virtually all of them are false. Here are some examples:
making love for the first time; having sex on Sunday; having sex
during your menstrual period; avoiding the full insertion of the
male's penis; taking a shower, douching, or doing calisthenics
afterward.

What's more, even among the legitimate techniques of birth

control, there are no foolproof methods. The fact is, there's only one sure way to avoid pregnancy: don't have sex.

Now that I'm pregnant, what should I do? I'm so confused.

It's important to realize that you don't have to do anything immediately. You have time to think about the options that are available to you. There's no need to rush into a decision you might regret later. You will want to consider carefully all the choices you have—marrying the father, keeping the baby, giving the baby for adoption. When an idea comes to you, take time to write it down and think about it. Then wait till tomorrow and see whether it still seems like a good idea. Talk to people in whom you have confidence, people who care about you. Spend time asking God what He would have you do in this situation. Although there are no Scripture verses that specifically give advice about this problem, the Bible is full of passages that provide God's principles for times when we need direction: Psalms 23; 32:8; 139:1-18; Isaiah 1:16-18; 40:11; 42:16; Jeremiah 29:11-13; 33:3; John 10:3, 4; 8:11; 16:13; Ephesians 5:15-17; and I John 1:9.

But the plans for my future will be all messed up. I want an abortion.

Tell me why you're considering that choice. (Be sensitive. Patiently listen to what the young woman has to say before you respond along the following lines.)

Abortion is a medical procedure that poses some risks for you. You must consider your health and long-term emotional and spiritual consequences such as guilt feelings. There is no "quick fix" possible in this circumstance.

More importantly, you must consider that now there is another life involved in this situation. You need to think about what is best for the baby as well as for yourself. (Chapter 6 provides further insight into the Biblical perspective on abortion.)

If I keep the baby, I'll have someone to love who will always love me.

It's true that keeping the baby is an option that is getting more and more popular. A mother develops a strong bond to the child she is carrying. But a baby is very different from a doll or a plaything. The child will grow up to be an independent person with a will of his or her own. This new person brings tension into the life of a parent, not just joy, love, and pleasure. You can probably see some of that in your own family.

Don't decide to keep your baby because of what the child can do for you. It's very important to ask yourself what will be best for the baby.

It's very natural to want a source of love at a lonely time like this. But no person can give you the kind of assurance and affection you desire—not your parents, your boyfriend, or even your baby. I'd like to suggest that you look to God. He never withholds His love. He cares for you so much that He sent His only Son to die for you.

I don't think I could stand to give my baby for adoption. It would be so hard!

Yes, it is a difficult thing to do. There is a lot of emotional pain anytime you give something that is part of you. This is a loss that must be mourned just like any other relationship that is broken through death or other circumstances.

If you choose adoption, you may want to be actively involved in the process. This will help you not to feel like a passive victim.

Many adoption agencies or people qualified to arrange private adoptions do all they can to involve the mother and/or father in the placement process if the birth parents wish to be involved. They may provide the birth parent with profiles of adoptive families from which he or she may select the couple most suited to raise the baby. The birth parent often can have information about the adoptive family but not their identity. Christian agencies will help you find adoptive families who are Christians also.

You will want those around you—parents, friends, counselors, agency staff, or people from your church—to support you and your decision. Sometimes you will cry because of this loss; other times you will need someone with whom you can share how it feels to be a mother whose child is cared for by others.

Remember that if you allow your child to be adopted, you are doing it because that is what would be best for the child, but, in the long run, it will also be best for you.

I can't tell my parents. My dad'll kill me!

This is a problem that can't be hidden from your parents.

Eventually they'll find out even if you don't tell them. It usually is best if you are the one who tells them.

Expect them to be surprised, maybe shocked. They may cry and they may be angry. The way they react at first may not show how they actually feel. Give them time to adjust to their feelings and get used to the idea that you are pregnant. Then you can begin working together on the best solution.

If you're really afraid of how your parents will react, another adult should be with you when you tell them—maybe your pastor or a friend's mother? If you want, I'll go with you. I can't make the decisions and it's not my place to break the news, but as a "neutral party," I can help keep the peace.

(If you sense the girl has any real fear for her physical safety, you should be sure that a third party is present and follows up the situation later.)

I told my parents I was pregnant, and they kicked me out of the house. What do I do now?

This is a tense time for all of you. If you have had a basically good relationship with your folks, it is likely that it will be restored soon. Give them time to get over their anger.

In the meantime, you need a place to stay. (Note: If the pregnant teen has no relatives nearby, contact area shelters or homes for women in difficult circumstances. There may also be a family in the church who would be willing to take her in for a while.)

Because you are on your own right now, be sure to take especially good care of yourself. You don't want to do anything that could harm you or the baby. That would include alcohol, tobacco, or any type of recreational drugs. See your family doctor or visit a clinic if you haven't already.

My boyfriend hardly speaks to me now. He never returns my calls, and he ignores me at school.

His attitude and behavior is wrong. Pregnancy takes two people, and the male and female have equal responsibility. Very likely your boyfriend is scared. Blaming you might be his way of avoiding feelings of guilt.

You both had a share in creating this pregnancy. But pregnancy can take the thrill out of a romantic relationship if that relationship was built mostly on sex. Even though it's painful to see this happening, it gives you a chance to re-examine this relationship to see if it's one you really want to continue.

I feel that people are pointing fingers at me, that they are talking behind my back. My reputation is ruined.

Reputations, like fashions, change. The important thing is that your value to God has not changed. Even though God was displeased with your actions, that did not affect His love for you. He is faithful!

Don't listen to the negative things people might be saying about you. Decide to get to know God better and do what He wants you to do. Soon you will feel better about yourself, and those who criticized you will realize that you want to do what is right.

But I know a lot of kids that are having sex. Why is God punishing me?

You're seeing a pretty dramatic example of the fact that actions have consequences. God has rules of right and wrong that don't depend on what the majority of people do. These rules are for our own good. Pregnancy is not a punishment. It's the natural consequence of sexual intercourse. Our bodies were designed to be able to reproduce.

The problem here is with timing—you got ahead of God's schedule by having sex, which resulted in a pregnancy, before you got married.

I don't want this to send me to hell.

God forgives us if we truly repent—say we are sorry, change our minds and go the opposite direction. It's essential to put faith and trust in Jesus Christ. All of us, you and me, are sinners (Rom. 3:23). And we *should* feel guilty when we sin, when we do things that displease God. Feelings of guilt are often like reminders that we need to ask His forgiveness. This forgiveness was provided for us through Christ's death on the Cross.

Good can come out of every situation—even this one. A new life, valuable to God and full of potential, has been created.

Maybe we should get married.

That's one option, but first you should analyze your relationship and whether you are really ready to get married. You wouldn't want to compound one mistake with a second that might lead to years of misery and/or divorce.

Before the pregnancy, what were the strengths and weaknesses of your relationship? Do you have a lot in common? What were your fights about? How have your feelings been changing toward one another now that you are pregnant? What would you like for the future? Is it possible to achieve?

Your relationship can go in several directions. You could decide to get married. You could break up altogether. You could stay single and, if you keep the baby, your boyfriend could give you support. Or you could decide to place your child for adoption and then live independently.

Don't take any drastic actions. There is no need to rush, and you want to avoid extra pressures and emotional challenges right now.

Try having discussions with your boyfriend that do not commit either of you to specific courses of action at first. Your relationship has entered a whole new phase, and you may feel you are seeing each other as strangers. Take the time to see how each other is reacting to the pregnancy. This wait-and-see period will help you make decisions later on.

There are legal aspects to consider as well. For example, if your boyfriend admits that he is the father of your child, he could become legally responsible for a portion of the costs of your pregnancy and, if you decide to keep the baby, for part of the child care costs as well.

Remember, though, that if your boyfriend declares he is the child's father and you accept this declaration, it is possible for him to have a voice in determining the child's future.

Sorting out the emotional, legal, and financial aspects of your relationship can be difficult, especially given the other pressures that you face. It may be helpful for you to work with a pastor or counselor or social worker on a regular basis until you have made the basic decisions in this area.

The Boyfriend's Questions and Concerns

I always thought a girl couldn't get pregnant if you made love standing up.

(Your response should be similar to question #2 that a pregnant teen might ask. See page 35.)

There are many myths about human sexuality and contraception. Now is not the time to be looking for foolproof birth control. Instead, try to learn God's view of sexuality and positive behaviors you can use to handle your sex drive. God created us as sexual beings; He sanctions the proper time for sex and reproduction: after marriage.

It's all her fault.

The girl is the one who carries the child, but procreation always takes two people. You are both responsible for this pregnancy. This is not the time for anyone to cast blame. (This is not true in the more rare cases of pregnancy resulting from rape or incest.)

The real problem is not pregnancy—it's sex outside of marriage. This is the time to think about correcting inappropriate behavior patterns; it is time to stop sexual activity until marriage.

Try to begin working together on solutions that will best benefit those involved. Whatever tensions were present in your relationship, they now are joined by the fact of this pregnancy. Try to cooperate with each other.

The other guys act like sex is no big deal.

Because of our culture and human biology, men and women have different views of sex. But however we approach the subject, there's no doubt that it's important. Intense emotions and potential life are involved—handle with care.

Love, mutual trust, and respect are vital. That's why God created the structure of marriage.

Also, God doesn't look at us in terms of whether we follow the crowd. He wants us as individuals to obey His rules—for our own good.

When she told me she was pregnant, we had a big fight. Now she won't even talk to me.

(Not all young men will try to evade responsibility. Some may want to be deeply involved with the decision making and will have strong opinions of what course of action to take. The mother, however, may shut out the father. She might be able to do this legally as well as emotionally.)

Given the changes that are taking place in her body as well as

41

in her life, you may sense mood swings which may make it hard for you to know how to relate to her. Be prepared to follow her lead and give her the emotional freedom to change her mind several times. This may be difficult for you to do because of your own emotional involvement. Ask God to give you patience during the difficult times and sensitivity to know when and how to support her.

This ruins all my plans.

It's true that the fact that your girlfriend is pregnant means some major adjustments; some things will have to change. But your whole life doesn't have to be in shambles. Ask yourself questions like these: What are my plans? What kind of priorities should I set? How can the situation of this pregnancy be used in a constructive way? Think through your answers to these questions, and ask God to guide you in this process.

I told her to get an abortion. It's not even human yet.

"It" really is human. Even very early in pregnancy, an independent life has begun. This life deserves the full consideration and respect of both mother and father since the child is unable to speak. (Offer a brief explanation of how life begins at conception.)

You both are in a joint situation. Do you think it is right at this point for one person to be issuing orders to the other? This is an intense, emotional time. Try to work together—if necessary, through a third party.

(Although the mother has many legal rights, she may be emotionally dominated by the boyfriend who could use his assumed authority to dictate to her. Be sensitive to this situation and intervene if necessary.)

I suppose we've got to get married now. It's the only decent thing to do.

Marriage is an option, but it's only one of the options. Don't choose it under pressure. It's a lifetime commitment—not a bandage for a problem. If you get married for the wrong reasons, you'll end up with a far worse problem. "Shotgun" weddings tend to backfire—teen marriages related to pregnancy have a higher divorce rate than the rest of society—which is plenty high already.

Consider: Would you get married now if she was not pregnant? How ready are you for marriage in terms of education and career?

The truth is, I don't love her. I don't even feel like I know her that well.

Remember, this time is an emotional roller-coaster. You're seeing each other in an entirely new light and under a new kind of pressure. That's a very different outlook from the one you had when you first met and started going out.

It's very likely that you *don't* know each other as well as you might. Young people often rush and put the physical aspect of a relationship ahead of all other steps.

Try to put aside the emotions and make clear-headed decisions that will serve you both—and the baby—over the long run.

What kind of say do I have in the baby's future?

Many legal rights are with the mother. However, the father is legally responsible for child care costs until the child is 18—if the mother decides to parent alone. This law, however, varies among states and is sporadically enforced.

Fathers who want to can ask to be a part of childbirth classes, and even help in delivery if both parties agree.

Questions and Comments from the Teen's Parents
We trusted her, and now look—she's betrayed us.

It is doubtful she'd do as drastic a thing as get pregnant just to defy or betray you. But right now, everybody is probably feeling betrayed. Hopes and plans are at risk. Remember, though, the one truly innocent party is the baby. Rather than point fingers, all sides should try to work together for his or her benefit.

Keep in mind—many girls who get pregnant are crying out for love and attention which they feel they have missed before. Try to fill that need as you work toward a solution of the pregnancy crisis.

How can we hold up our heads in this town?

Pregnancy is not a sin. Life is a gift from God. The focus of anger should not be on the pregnancy, but rather on the conduct—sex outside of marriage—that brought it about. However, don't judge the sinner; we're all guilty. It just happens that pregnancy reflects in a very public way sin that is similar to what we all experience.

Let's look to God for approval, not to our reputation or prestige in the eyes of the world. Find out His plan for this crisis and obey it.

I'm too young to be a grandparent!

It's natural to feel shock. This is not the storybook way to become grandparents. It's out of sequence.

Understand, though, that new life is a natural part of the human cycle. Accept the fact that your family is being reorganized into new relationships. Let the dust settle. It will take time to work into the new mold, but it can be done.

What can we say to our other children?

Relate the situation to things your kids already have experienced. This is no different (in terms of action and consequences) than failing to do homework for a course in school. Sometimes you think you can get by without anyone knowing, but a surprise exam can find you out. The lesson here is to follow the rules (in the case of sexual activity, it means following God's rules), think ahead, and prepare to accept the consequences of your actions.

There is, however, one difference between the example of failing to be prepared for classes and pregnancy. Pregnancy results in something good—a human life. The timing was wrong and the situation may be very complex, but the question is, how will you as a family base your upcoming decisions? This is a good time to work together, with no judgment of your pregnant daughter, in helping her think ahead and accept the results of her conduct.

This may also be a good time to broach the subject of sex education with your younger children.

Since this happened, all our family does is fight.

Take a step back and reappraise the situation. A crisis like this usually brings to the surface many older, unrelated tensions and problems. Try to separate them from the issue at hand.

Remember that every member of the family has a stake in the outcome of the problem. All should work together. Consider bringing in an understanding, "neutral" party to help you sort out the various questions and concerns.

My husband's not talking to anyone, not even to me.

As grandparents, you both probably feel frustrated at having to be "responsible" for actions you did not commit and which you don't condone. In such a situation it is common for people to express that frustration in anger or withdrawal. However, don't let this situation go on too long. It will be helpful for you to see a counselor.

I want her out of the house, and to be honest, I don't care what she does or where she goes.

Will this make the problem go away? It might worsen things considerably. Your daughter needs you now. She might seem defiant and angry, but really she is desperate. Try to rise above your emotions and address the long-term needs here.

She's got to get an abortion. I want a quick solution to this problem.

There are no quick fixes. Abortion is a medical procedure and it poses risks. Just like the decision to engage in sex before marriage, abortion has its consequences, too. Now is a good time to model for your children how to anticipate consequences before taking action. There are the long-term emotional and spiritual consequences to abortion. Also, abortion is not condoned by biblical teachings.

You must realize that your daughter has to make her own decisions. You can advise, suggest, and help her work through various options, but she has to take responsibility. That will be best for her—and for you.

Of course they're getting married. The two of them caused this problem, and now they have to live with the consequences.

Marriage should not be a penalty. If it is wrong, then two wrongs won't make a right. Marriage must be entered into willingly and with mutual love and respect.

A generation ago, "shotgun" weddings were one of the few options available to pregnant teens. Now there is far less pressure; there is no need to feel locked into it.

Also—try to view the baby as a separate person, worthy of full human dignity. The consequence of this misconduct is the *crisis* that the pregnancy causes. However, the baby is not the "bad result"; he or she is an innocent person.

She's keeping that child. Our family doesn't give away its own flesh and blood.

I think it's good you have a strong sense of family loyalty. This will be an asset as you work together toward a solution. On the other hand, don't let a notion of family obligations imprison you.

Use your closeness to support one another—even if this means "losing" a member of the family—the child. Remember, it may be best for both the child and your daughter if you consider adoption.

I think she should give the child for adoption. It's the fairest way for all concerned.

I'm glad you want to be fair. This is the kind of family problem that often divides relatives into factions. If you look out for one another's needs, everyone will benefit.

Adoption is an option. But remember, teenage mothers today are under far less social stigma. She may want to consider the possibility of keeping the child. The word you used— "give"—suggests a sense of loss. And it's true that she will "lose" the child in the sense of not being with him or her during all the growing-up years. This may be the best solution for all parties, even if it is painful. But don't be hasty. Consider all the possibilities.

It's all right. We'll take over. Her mother and I will raise this child.

It's good that you want to be involved in your daughter's pregnancy. I'm always saddened when something like this drives parents and their children apart. You're off to a good start in working with one another.

Still, it may not be best for you to take over. That's a natural reaction for parents—to want to come in, pick up the pieces, and make everything "right" for their kids. But, unfortunately, you can't make everything right in a situation like this.

You've already raised a family. This child is your daughter's.

She will have to take responsibility—in order for her to continue growing up, and because your grandchild needs decisions to come from the mother, even if that means releasing the child for adoption.

Try to let the new relationships grow. You're grandparents now, which means leaving the day-to-day authority with your daughter. Of course, you still can advise her and support her.

Our family just can't afford what this child will cost.

I can understand your nervousness about finances. But don't let money dictate whether the child should be kept or given for adoption.

If your daughter really wants to be a single parent and is prepared for all the duties that are involved, help is available. There are government programs for help with clothing and food, as well as medical care. If she plans carefully, she can even continue her education and work toward getting a good job. All this will take discipline on her part—and resourcefulness in looking for assistance. But it can be done. So try to keep a realistic view of money, but don't let it dominate your thinking as decisions are made.

Our daughter wants to keep the child. But marriage to the father is out of the question. What kind of male role model will the child have?

It's very important for the development of the child to include a male role model. There are a range of options.

You, as grandfather, might be one of them. Will the child have uncles who can help? Also, consider the Big Brother program through schools and the YMCA. This is a program that puts older teenagers and college students in touch with younger children. They meet socially on an informal basis for sports, a movie or just to talk. An activity like this will put this child in touch with other adults.

If possible, your daughter should consider maintaining a relationship with the father—if only for the child's sake. The child will care deeply about his or her father, and any link will be helpful.

You say we should treat our daughter as an adult and let her make her own decisions, but we're the ones who are taking care of her, and she's a minor—so we're legally responsible for her.

You've pinpointed one of the most frustrating aspects of this situation. There is no easy solution, but as grandparents you can create a framework in which your daughter can safely grow to greater maturity and independence.

Set limits with love. You're still well within your rights to give her guidelines on dating, school, and spending money. At the same time, she should begin to make her own decisions in matters such as education and career. Your job is to see that she keeps on track.

Also, you should make sure the basics are covered—shelter, medical care, insurance, etc. This does not obligate you to care for your daughter the rest of your lives. Instead, you should work toward encouraging her to become more and more independent. Be honest with yourselves about the amount of help your daughter should have,

To get the ball rolling, try giving her some basic duties—help around the house, etc. Help her set realistic goals she can meet on a daily basis. Reward her when she accomplishes a goal. This will help her become more self-sufficient.

Questions/Comments from the Church

I can't see how this could happen to a good Christian family.

It can happen to anyone. All of us face temptation, and all of us give in at certain points.

Remember the example of King David? He was a man after God's own heart, yet he fell into sexual sin. We're all vulnerable, and we can't claim any special "goodness" as a protection. The only real protection is God's grace. With it, we can build a better defense system, but if that system fails, God expects us to hold one another up.

The two families were such close friends. Now they're not speaking. This could divide the whole congregation.

That's a real danger. The best solution is not to take sides. If possible, the families should work together with a "neutral" party, such as a social worker or counselor. Other people should be supportive and maintain any personal friendships with members of the families.

How can we show love without seeming to condone the sin?

This can be done by focusing on two parts of this situation. The sin here was sex outside of marriage. God has clear rules on this subject, which we are not to take lightly or break. Nevertheless, we also should not judge others in the sense of delivering a penalty by withholding our love.

Love should be shown to the parties involved. Communicate a sense of forgiveness—it may encourage them to forgive each another. Also, see the life of the child as cause for rejoicing. God has a specific plan for each life. In our limited view, this may not be the ideal way to begin a life, but God can redeem the situation and use this young person for His glory.

Remember, God's love is unconditional. Christ loved us and died for us while we were sinners, and His grace can overcome this problem—if we all submit to Him.

For the parties involved, emphasize small, practical outlets rather than philosophical discussions. Keep in touch through cards and telephone calls. Give baby clothes, a shower, offers of transportation to medical appointments. Make it known you are available to help, but don't intrude.

I don't want to see her kicked out of church, but isn't some kind of discipline needed here?

We have to maintain clear standards. Involve the pastor at this point if disciplinary action is called for. Make it clear that we will not tolerate sex outside of marriage—which refers to all people, not just teens who happen to get pregnant.

A lot depends on the young mother's attitude. If she is defiant or hostile, it may be necessary to ask her (and the father, if he is in the church) to step down from leadership positions within the church. If she shows signs of repentance and a desire to continue her fellowship, that should be honored. This a prime time to demonstrate the meaning of God's forgiveness.

And in all cases, the fact of pregnancy must not be condemned. This is a natural bodily function—and it involves the life of an innocent party.

That young man needs some serious talking to.

There should be no sniping at him from the sidelines. Your approach will be modeled on that for the mother—much depends upon his attitude toward the situation.

Too often the father's role in pregnancy is either ignored or made the focus of great anger. Both approaches are wrong. This is a confused young man, who needs counseling and practical advice (legal, educational, vocational). The conception of a child is an irrevocable act, but forgiveness and restoration are always available.

I just don't see how she's going to fit in anymore.

The structure of our church fellowship shouldn't be so rigid that people with new needs can't find a place.

Think of a church as a hospital, where hurting people can be helped. When a person comes into a hospital, there is an immediate assessment of the person's needs. He or she is sent to a place in the hospital where the appropriate help is available: emergency room, long-term care, outpatient, surgery. So, too, the different groups in our church have things to offer this woman—spiritual help from the deacons, companionship from the young adults group, financial help from the stewards, etc. It's our job to adjust to meet her various needs.

She's a "bad apple." I don't want her to influence the rest of the kids.

In most cases, her problems are so evident that no one will want to copy her. If you do not fawn over her or give her "red carpet" treatment, watching her go through the process of dealing with this problem may be an excellent object lesson for other young people in the congregation.

What the other kids need to see is that problems don't come with built-in happy endings; it takes hard work and tears before problems are resolved—and even then there may be no perfectly desirable answer. But God can work good through this. He provides grace in daily problems. One of the primary avenues of grace will be the church's care, and it will be very important for the youth to see this in action, too.

All the other kids are talking about her.

Gossip must stop. Meet with the people who are doing the gossiping—either as individuals or as a group.

The goal here is to discuss facts—in a calm, dispassionate manner.

The church should rally around the girl and show support. Be glad she's not dropping out of the congregation. Be glad she is carrying her baby to term. This is a courageous decision, given our society's pressure to have an abortion and the easy access to this procedure.

If it happened to her, it can happen to anyone. What's to stop this from becoming an epidemic?

Teens are under a lot of pressure to get involved in sex—and that includes Christian teens. As adults, we can't spy on them, and it won't work to make grand pronouncements.

As a congregation, we have to identify the "pressure points" at which the world encourages teen sex and show God's answer. For example—teens have sex because they feel a lack of personal self-esteem; because they don't have personal goals; because they crave the acceptance of their peers. But God is our true supply for these needs.

This threatens the witness of our church to the entire community.

You may be right. Credibility can be a problem in some situations. But the issue is not "How could one of *our* members get pregnant?" It should be no surprise that a church is made up of sinners who need to be forgiven. If our witness to the community has said something different, then we're in trouble for *that* reason.

Rather, the issue here is, "How do we treat this young woman?" Think of the pious hypocrisy of the congregation in Hawthorne's novel, *The Scarlet Letter.* They shunned a single mother and made her life miserable. The community will judge us on how we treat this young mother. If we show her love and offer practical solutions—while making it clear that we adhere to God's principles—our witness, not to mention her life, will be all the stronger.

I want to help, but I'm afraid they'll think I'm nosy, just butting in.

A lot depends on your relationship with the family prior to this problem. Are they open to sharing their needs with you? If so, don't shut them out. Once they are certain you are available to help, let them call the shots. No doubt their moods will change over time, and in some circumstances they will welcome help and in other cases they'll want privacy. You should keep a flexible attitude and allow them to have these shifts.

I know the girl's parents. They're not saying much, but I can tell they're not coping well. How can we help?

If the family members are withdrawing into themselves, we need to set up a liaison between them and the church. This can be a friend, like you, or a professional—such as a counselor. Different people prefer a different approach—the warmth and familiarity of a friend, or the more detached and professional relationship with a counselor. We as a congregation must be sensitive to their wishes.

What we can do is to make it known to them what services are available: day care, clothing, help with finances, etc. To a large extent, we should follow the family's lead. When they initiate contact, we can respond. But they need to feel free in coming forward. Then we can respond in love.

CHAPTER FOUR

COUNSELING THE PREGNANT TEEN

OFTEN, THE PERSON MOST UPSET OVER TEENAGE PREGNANCY is the individual who is called upon to give help. Of course, the expectant mother is apprehensive and full of questions, but she's young. You, however, have a fuller sense of what teen pregnancy implies. And that can be frightening.

The condition involves three generations of people: the infant, the young parents, and, often, the stunned grandparents. Each has distinct but interrelated needs. Teen pregnancy affects virtually every aspect of life: health, finances, education, career, spirituality, sexuality, and individual and family goals. It's a nationwide phenomenon yet an intensely personal problem. And, suddenly, it's touched your life.

This chapter reviews sound counseling techniques for use in a situation involving a crisis pregnancy. It puts the fundamental principles of modern counseling into a Christian context, with advice for how people in a counseling role can both maintain their own equilibrium and provide the best possible advice for the pregnant teen.

There are as many options for involvement with a pregnant teenager as there are individual cases. The pregnant teen may be your daughter, the friend of your daughter, the daughter of your friend. She may be a neighbor, an employee, a member of your church or Sunday school class. You may have known her since she was a child, or you might have met only after this crisis engulfed her. You may be close in age or a generation or two older. But somehow you feel some reason to assist her at this time.

If you are a man, the ideal situation is to transfer the case to a woman. If it is not possible to transfer the case, be sure to involve a woman (preferably a mother) as a team member with you in the counseling process. But bear in mind that two helpers can be awkward and make it difficult for the teen to establish rapport with either. It is best to make this transition immediately because, not only will the new mother need the assurance and insight of a woman, but you will need her objectivity. In most cases, crisis pregnancies occur partially as an attempt to fill an intimacy vacuum. That vacuum probably still exists, and one counseling task will be to address it and guide the young mother to the Lord and His plan for filling it. However, do not think that you are immune from the temptation to fill it inappropriately. Having a woman partner present will reduce this temptation and will relieve the tension of talking about intimate matters.

As you contemplate getting involved with the needs of a pregnant teenager, evaluate the situation. Primarily, the young mother needs a sense of consistency and commitment. You don't have to be and do all things for her. But you must know what you can offer, and you should extend that offer in clear terms. Consider the following questions to clarify your own motives and resources:

• How well do you know this young woman?
• Has she approached you for help? If so, what has she requested?
• What can you offer? Time? Friendship? Medical or legal assistance? Financial help? Clothing and supplies? A place to stay? A job?
• Why do you want to help her?
• Have you or someone you know experienced a similar crisis?
• How does your schedule look for the next year (the length of time she will likely need a strong support system)?

Be wary of a desire to "straighten out her life." It's not your right, and it's unrealistic to insist on plans that the young woman will not accept. Your personalities do not have to mesh exactly, but there should be mutual respect. If you know other members of the young woman's family, you may want to discuss with them any involvement you might have in the situation. Legally, you might not need their permission to assist the mother, but this is a stressful time for everyone, and you would do well to cultivate a sense of harmony.

What does your own family think about your involvement? Are they concerned or upset about the time it will take from them? Are there problems or areas of stress at home that need your attention? Ministry to a teenage mother is not the way to resolve your own hurts and needs. The main reason you want to help this young woman should *not* be to "make up" for problems—real or imagined—in your own life. Be sure you can deliver what you offer. It's better simply to drive a girl to her medical appointments on a consistent basis than to make promises you cannot keep.

Above all, it's not necessary for you to carry this problem alone. That's probably the first worthwhile advice that a pregnant teenager hears, but it's equally true for her helpers. Teen pregnancy is a lengthy, multifaceted problem. To reach genuine solutions, it's essential for everyone involved to avoid burnout. Today, more than ever, there are qualified professionals and laypeople who can form a network with the families and friends of a pregnant teen. In many communities a full range of services is available to help. Many of these services have a Christian perspective. Not all of them can be found under one roof, and it may take some work to find them or to develop your own organization, but results can make the effort worthwhile.

Yet, even while ministry to women in crisis pregnancy becomes more professional and extensive, there remains need for the individual who feels nudged by God to give specific help to a particular teenager. Your personal input could be what makes the difference. If you feel that leading, follow it. Historically, this has been the basis of Christian service. The task may seem overwhelming, but that's the time to remember one of the names given to the Messiah, Jesus Christ: "Wonderful Counselor." His expertise can guide you through any situation.

The Purpose of Counseling

Whether you provide basic items to the young mother (such as maternity clothes) or offer advice on a wider range of topics, remember that your role is not to make decisions or set policy. Rather, you must create an atmosphere of trust and helpfulness that allows the woman to make her own choices. Any "arm-twisting" that you attempt may hopelessly compromise your relationship. Also try to avoid a common tendency to become an emotional rescuer. Present options to the mother, helping her to weigh the pros and cons.

Know Your Authority

Counseling is an opportunity for service. God wants to work through you, and the pregnant woman looks to you, because you have something to offer. It may be your professional expertise or a sense of empathy and caring. You should feel free to say what you think, based upon reliable evidence, and present it as an option for the mother to consider.

There is a time for firmness. For example, research confirms that smoking and use of illicit drugs can greatly harm the infant; you can lovingly but clearly make this point. On the other hand, the Bible does not provide a uniform, straightforward, clear answer as to whether a woman should marry the father of her child, keep or place the baby for adoption. You can examine Scripture with the woman and evaluate the various implications of her case, but it is not appropriate to become dogmatic about these issues.

Building a Solid Relationship

You don't have to be a professional counselor to establish practical rapport with someone in need. Try to cultivate the following characteristics in yourself:

1. Unconditional acceptance—You must be able to accept the woman as a worthwhile individual. You needn't approve of her life-style, but you must not condemn her because of her problem. Keep in mind that Christ loved us while we were unrepenting sinners, and His mercy covers the sins we continue to commit.

2. Empathy—You need to understand what the woman feels and demonstrate this fact to her while retaining enough detachment to give practical advice and assistance. Don't look at her as merely one more "case" to be helped, but don't become so emotionally wrapped up in her troubles that you lose objectivity.

3. Sincerity—You're human, too, and don't be afraid to show it. In the long run, the woman will appreciate knowing that you had to struggle alongside her to meet her needs. This is preferable to acting aloof or pretending to know all the answers.

The Skills of Counseling

"Communication" is a popular concept today, and many studies analyze its components by scientific research. Experts will tell you, for example, of the impact that each of the following variables has in the accurate transmission of a message: spoken word, gestures and body posture, and tone of voice. But rather than weigh you down with statistics, it seems better to focus on some useful, common-sense techniques recommended by the Christian Action Council:

Restatement. One of the best ways to show a person your interest in her thoughts is to rephrase them. This indicates that you are paying attention, and it will give the woman opportunity to confirm that you have understood her correctly. Mutual understanding leads to trust. Don't repeat, parrot-like, everything the woman says. But when you sense she has made a major point or declaration of her feelings, you can use this technique as a method of summarizing what has been discussed.

Interpretive Listening. Sometimes a person's full message does not come out in words. "Body language," tone of voice, and certain figures of speech are ways that people use to express themselves. Think of the many shades of meaning you can give to the statement, "I'm so glad to be here." It may be a literal statement of fact. Spoken in a sarcastic tone, the words might mean just the opposite; they also can convey relief, hesitation, or other emotions.

Interpretive listening will help you decipher the fuller meaning of what a person says. But you always want to test the accuracy of your analysis, so you need to follow up your interpretation with restatement. It's best to use a qualifying phrase to begin your restatement, so as not to put words into the woman's mouth. (Woman: "My mom always paid more attention to my little sister. I guess that's because she's smarter and prettier than I am." Counselor: "It sounds like you're hurt because your mother didn't give you all the love you wanted.")

Good Questions. These queries are open-ended, designed to help the person verbalize feelings and emotions. The questions should not be structured so they require simple yes/no responses or begin with "why," since that implies judgment.

Avoid asking questions too rapidly; you want a conversation, not an interrogation. Allow time for the person to think about the question and formulate a response. Refrain from sneaking your opinion into the question ("You are going to keep the baby, aren't you?"). Some examples of good questions: "How do you feel about your pregnancy?" "What events led you to break up with the father?" "What would you like in a living arrangement during your pregnancy?"

Feedback. This technique lets you inform the person how you think the conversation is going. It's a way to help the person set a new direction for your talk if you believe things are not going well; it's also an encouragement for a positive line of conversation. To keep your remarks non-threatening, make the focus of what you say "I," not "you." Feedback comes in three parts: "I feel (response) when you (words or behavior), because (reason)." For example: "I feel hurt when you talk sarcastically, because you don't seem to realize I want to help you with this budget." This is preferable to "You're always so sarcastic. How do you expect me to help you?"

Confrontation. Many secular counselors now reject the tool of confrontation because they accept no objective basis of right and wrong from which to take a position. As Christians, however, we can look to the Bible as giving an absolute standard of truth. Keep in mind, though, that the Bible challenges *all* of us to conform to God's will. You are as subject to God's authority as the people you counsel.

When you base your position on Scripture, you have the right—indeed, the duty—to tell the person the truth about her perceptions or conduct and urge her to conform them to God's criteria. The prophet Nathan confronted King David quite bluntly about his adulterous relationship with Bathsheba. Psalm 51 is David's response, a powerful expression of God's power to redeem the worst situations:

Create in me a pure heart, O God, and renew a steadfast spirit within me. Do not cast me from your presence or take your Holy Spirit from me. Restore to me the joy of your salvation and grant me a willing spirit, to sustain me. Then I will teach transgressors your ways, and sinners will turn back to you (Ps. 51:10-13, RSV).

Confrontation is a powerful tool and must be used carefully. It must be rooted in your love for the person, not in scorn or a sense of superiority. Don't aim to condemn, but carefully and clearly point the way toward lasting benefits. You should use confrontation only when you already have established a trusting relationship. The truth, as you speak it, may be hard for the person to bear, but practical good can result when the person realizes you have her welfare as your motivation.

When using confrontation, keep it specific. Avoid sweeping generalities. Try to pinpoint the area in the person's life where change is both necessary and attainable. ("I want you to stop using that profane language to talk about your stepfather. It can only make your relationship worse.") Later you can go on to more deeply rooted problems. When the subject of your confrontation has been resolved, move forward from there. Don't linger over old issues. Use confrontation judiciously, and be sure it never becomes the focal point of your talks.

Today's Options

Teen pregnancy has existed as long as there have been teenagers. But until the last decade, many efforts to help this situation were not always positive.

It used to be a time for panic. A shotgun wedding, a quickly arranged "visit" to a distant aunt, adoption via a friendly lawyer, a back-alley abortion, or having the baby raised by relatives —these were the traditional means of coping with a teen pregnancy. The idea was to make everything go as quickly and as neatly as possible.

Bev O'Brien, á homemaker in Omaha, Nebraska, assumed this same urgency would prevail when she learned her unmarried 19-year-old daughter was expecting a child. But as she writes in *Mom . . . I'm Pregnant*, she found a vastly different situation than had been common when she was young:

While the heartbreak [of a crisis pregnancy] hasn't changed, it seems that almost everything else has.

Maybe we've learned to become more honest in our appraisal of ourselves, and less likely to judge others. Or we've seen so many types of behavior via public media that we've become unshockable. Or we are better educated regarding the hidden factors behind the unwed pregnancy.

Whatever the reason, one thing is certain: the outlook for today's unwed mother is far more positive than it used to be.

Support replaces criticism. Calmness overrules panic. Once, the unwed pregnancy gave rise to hasty decisions, arrived at in an emotionally charged atmosphere and aggravated by an extreme sense of urgency. Uppermost in everyone's mind was how to cover up the girl's error.

Today the question is, "How do we discover what is best for this girl's potential?" [1]

As you counsel those involved with a crisis pregnancy, you can help them unfold their many options. Together, you can see the redemption of a serious problem. It can become a time of growth and personal development.

Sorting It All Out

The people who approach you about a crisis pregnancy almost always will be in a panic. It's a frightening, highly emotional time. Your first objective is to quell their anxiety. True, the stakes are high, but the outcome is not preordained to be negative. There are as many opportunities in this time as there are risks.

Crisis pregnancy can even be one of the more manageable types of trauma. Consider: Catastrophic illness, divorce, or the loss of a job have no clear-cut time schedule; their effects can drag on for years without resolution. Pregnancy, on the other hand, has a very specific timetable. Its symptoms and complications are well known. Without minimizing the problem, this does help keep things in perspective. When counseling a person in crisis, break the problem into "digestible" segments. Set priorities. Draw up a calendar of things that must be done.

At your first meeting, compile a list of all the things the young woman fears and another of what she needs. The lists may be lengthy, but they do set "boundaries" around the problem. Now rank the items. For example, fears that the baby may be deformed should not preoccupy a woman who has missed her first period. Set that worry aside until later.

What are the first-line items to be addressed? You need to deal with the following right away:

1. *Abuse.* Is the woman at risk for sexual, physical, or emotional harassment? If so, she will need a safe place to stay, certainly for the present, perhaps for her entire pregnancy.

2. *Chemical dependency.* Does she have problems with alcohol, smoking, or illicit drugs? Prompt treatment is the only way to avoid lasting harm for herself and the child.

3. *Living expenses.* If her boyfriend or parents have kicked her out, she will need assistance with food and housing.

4. *Health care.* Does she have a doctor? The sooner she can begin prenatal treatment, the better for herself and the baby.

Other problems are not as pressing. Overall finances may be less of an emergency than she thinks. Insurance, public assistance, Medicaid, food stamps, and private grants are available. Many hospitals will extend payment schedules for women in financial need. Maternity clothes often are available at the Salvation Army or Goodwill stores.

As a way to balance the lists of needs and worries, ask the young woman to note her various assets. She might have skills from a summer job, a good relationship with parents or a special friend. She might have some money saved or a clear idea of her vocational goals. This list won't make her problems go away, but it can show a frightened girl that she is not alone or without resources.

Decision-making Skills

Now that you have documented the problems, fears, and resources of this crisis, introduce coping strategies. Again, "know thyself" is the rule. Help the woman assess her method of making decisions.

Ask her to think back to other "crossroad" experiences in her life. The death of a grandparent, enrolling at a new school, starting a hobby—all are examples. How did she cope? Ask her to compare her previous coping techniques with her approach to the current problem. Does she blame others for her problems? Is she impulsive? Does she demand instant solutions? Will she take risks? Overall, is she an optimist or a pessimist? Does she expect others to make decisions for her? Is she a perfectionist?

These questions may sound basic to an adult, but they are by no means certain to a teen just coming to grips with her own personality in the midst of a major crisis.

Handbook for Pregnant Teenagers, by Linda Roggow and Carolyn Owen, points out that good decisions come from the following steps:

1. Identify the problem.
2. List alternative courses of action.
3. Gather relevant information.
4. Weigh the consequences of each alternative.
5. Know the risks.
6. Measure each alternative against your personal values.
7. Make the decision that is best for you. [2]

Pregnant teens need special help in dealing with the pressure that comes from other people. The young woman may have a deep sense of shame and regret, which makes her especially vulnerable to following the wishes of others against her better judgment and self-interest. Her parents, friends, the father of her child, and many others can bring inappropriate pressure. The young mother cannot ignore these people, but she must not let them manage her life. Much of your work as counselor may be at the diplomatic level, helping to keep peace among the various parties, while giving the mother "space" to make decisions that are best for her as an individual.

People rarely are ambivalent about unwed pregnancy, and the mother probably will get an earful from those around her: "You've got to get an abortion. A baby would tie you down for the rest of your life." "You're going to raise that child yourself. No one in this family gives away their own flesh and blood." "Place the child for adoption—it's the only way she'll have a decent life." Encourage the girl to resist manipulation. The Bible makes it clear that God has a specific purpose for each individual on earth. But unlike some people, He never forces obedience. The mother, assuming she is a Christian, can discern God's plan by noting the wise opinions of others, searching the Bible, and praying.

Future Shock

Teens have, at best, an erratic sense of the future. They'll fail to use birth control because they don't connect the act of sexual intercourse with what happens nine months later. They keep their infants or place them for adoption with little regard for long-term consequences. "It seemed okay at the time" is a byword among adolescents. It's not really their fault; they simply lack the maturity of adults. But pregnancy forces a teen into the adult world. She has to make life-and-death decisions about a child, and she must consider what pregnancy means to the future of her own health.

Help her set goals. What would she like for an education? High school diploma or equivalency degree? College? Right now, finishing ninth or tenth grade might be her loftiest ambition. Help her to see how education ties into a career and financial stability. Does she want to work? Professionally or part time? Does she have a vocational field of interest? Would she like to remain single when she is an adult? Marry? Have a family? You can't expect a teen to map an entire life's plan at this time, but you can expose her to the range of options that are available. If she can set any clear goals for her education or career, she will find it easier to make decisions that will lead to those goals.

Values Are Variable

What does she believe in? Does she have any idea? Part of the quagmire of teen pregnancy is that the young woman often lacks a clear sense of direction. By guiding (not brainwashing), you can expose her to the security of self-knowledge, of making a commitment to beliefs that she understands.

Probably this teen has accumulated a grab bag of notions from family and friends, television, religious training, and personal experience. Don't be surprised that these values may be contradictory, incomplete, and subject to change at virtually a moment's notice.

Help the young woman to recognize the difference between internal and external values. The former represent those values to which she has a personal commitment, for which she will make sacrifices and around which she should base her decisions. Even when the odds are stacked against her, she really believes in these values. Paradoxically, though, external values may seem more important at first. They come from other people. She endorses them because it seems the thing to do; she is afraid of rejection if she goes against them. Many times a teenage girl agrees to sexual intercourse with a boy she cares about rather than risk losing him by refusing. When questioned about what sex means to her or what benefit she derives from it, she will have little to say.

It won't do much good to talk to a pregnant girl about values in the theoretical sense. But by speaking in practical terms, you can give the subject a real-world application. How does she view the changes in her body? Does she consider herself to be carrying a child? Why or why not? What kind of life does she imagine would be best for the child? A traditional home with parents? A single-parent arrangement? How important does she think it is for the child and father to know each other? What type of life would she like to see the child have? Education? Career?

Many teens have clear ideas on such subjects, and by drawing them out in conversation, you can help the teens set and pursue goals. As values begin to align into a consistent pattern, decision making becomes easier since some options will be inappropriate when compared to the values that have been defined. For example, a mother who wrestles with not wanting to marry the father but who believes her child needs a two-parent home may be helped by learning how single mothers and their children function. If the woman sees that single mothers can be successful parents, her anxiety about enduring an undesired marriage may be reduced, or this goal-setting process may help her realize that adoption may be the best choice for the child.

A Method for the Motives

As a counterpart to helping a pregnant teen identify her values, talk with her about why she wants to pursue a certain course of action. As we all know, it's possible to conjure up an exalted justification for any type of conduct. It's even possible to do the right thing for the wrong reasons, and vice versa.

Help the girl to see that, however justified her antipathy toward certain people, she should not make decisions in a reactive manner: to win pity, for revenge, to hurt someone, out of jealousy. A girl who wants to keep her child so "there will always be someone to love me" will face disappointment. But a young woman who elects to keep the child because she has the determination and self-confidence to carry out the task has a far better chance for success. Teens who keep their children out of a desire to force the child's father into marriage, to "keep up" with their friends, or to gain "independent/adult" status will not be successful parents. Similar examples could be cited for the other options a young mother may undertake.

Emotions Are Okay

Don't expect most discourses with an unwed mother to be calm. A crisis such as this brings out many deeply held feelings. People also use these times to vent hostility that is not related to the problem. As counselor, you must referee. People need freedom to express feelings, but not to the point of hurting one another or making the difficult situation even worse.

Also keep in mind that serving as a counselor does not make you a doormat. The people you help will respect you more if you set fair limits. You don't need telephone calls late at night unless there is an emergency of epic proportion. You do need time off for your own work, family, and personal goals.

While you work with people, be sure that everyone's emotions remain under control. A few ill-timed words can have devastating results. Set ground rules: no name calling; everyone gets a turn to speak without interruption; participants must agree to a common goal of finding out what is best for all parties involved—for the mother and child first of all, then for the others.

Presenting the Gospel

Crisis pregnancies provide a unique time for witnessing the truth of Christianity. But you must handle the situation with respect for the individuals involved and without manipulation.

In essence, the entire message of the Bible is how God can transform bad situations into good ones. This work of restoration was the reason Christ came to earth. Innocent of sin, He chose to accept the punishment we deserve. This opens the way to reconciliation with God. We need to accept this as completed fact. It gives us an eternal life with God and a new avenue to practical, divine wisdom for facing life. That is "Good News" indeed for a teen caught in a crisis pregnancy.

At the same time, you never should demand that a person accept these beliefs before you are willing and available to provide help. And you should not present the Gospel only in terms of "Jesus will make you feel better." It's true, knowing the love and power of Christ brings great joy, but Jesus is not a panacea. He is Lord of all creation. Everyone must be willing to accept Christ's authority as well as His love and forgiveness.

Loss of personal dignity is a common element in unwed pregnancy. The woman who suffers rape or incest feels violated. The young teen who is pressured into having sex to "prove" her love has been manipulated. The ghetto resident for whom school seems useless and a good job unattainable may choose to get pregnant out of boredom or despair.

These women need practical assistance, of course. But decades of social action programs have shown that you can't solve problems with money alone. The lack of dignity and purpose these women feel represents an extreme form of what all of us experience: the need to be loved, to be sure our lives count for something. Only one answer can satisfy that yearning—realizing and experiencing the unconditional love of God. The security of Christ's love can give a woman the resolve to go on and handle her problems with His help.

It is also important to show the practical side of your faith. The pregnant teen has more on her mind than her relationship to God. But you can show her Biblical examples that are relevant to her circumstances. For example, Moses' mother was unable to keep her infant son, and released him into the care of Pharaoh's daughter, trusting God to take care of him through her. He wound up as one of the greatest leaders in history.

Concentrate on showing your faith more than telling it. Many teens are suspicious and hostile at first toward the people who want to help them. If you can demonstrate genuine Christian concern, your actions will be convincing. Then, at the right time, you can explain Bible verses that prompt your actions.

Weighing the Choices

These general principles will help in a wide range of counseling situations. Now it is time to address the major options that confront a pregnant teenager.

Abortion—This is not a helpful or legitimate solution for the problem of crisis pregnancy. The Bible does not sanction abortion. It offers no situation, commandments, or sayings that would justify abortion except when the life of the mother is in danger. Later (in chapter six) we'll review the numerous references in the Judaeo-Christian tradition that support the sanctity of human life.

Nevertheless, a pregnant teen may think of abortion first. In many cases, the underlying reason is desperation—the fear that no other course of action is as available or simple. You, however, can demonstrate that many avenues are open which serve the interests of both mother and child.

You should never use the deception of implying that you support abortion or would help a girl get one with the hope that you can talk her out of it later. It is both morally wrong and unnecessary to lie about your position.

On the other hand, don't get into an argument with the young mother over abortion. Instead, keep asking questions (such as: "May I ask why you are interested in having an abortion?") that help her reach her own conclusions. As she gives her reasons, you will have opportunity to show how other alternatives are available. Do not force her into any course of action. Help her to think for herself. "Do you know how abortions are performed?" "Has someone talked with you about the possible complications from an abortion?" "Do you think abortion would solve your problem?"

You want to help an expectant mother to regard her fetus as a person, not as a problem. If a woman does not believe she carries another human life within her, she will view pregnancy as she would an unsightly mole—a nuisance to be rid of.

Some supporters of the pro-life movement attempt to frighten women away from abortion by showing them pictures of aborted infants. These pictures are an appalling document of what abortion does. They deserve to be seen by policymakers and citizens. But we must not use them to horrify a pregnant woman. An equally effective and far more positive approach is to show pictures of the development of human life within the womb. Prenatal photography gives elegant, winsome views of the fetus, clearly showing its human form. These images offer dramatic evidence that the child who to be delivered at nine months is the same essential person he or she was at six months and six weeks.

Motherhood—The teen who decides against abortion will be a mother for at least nine months, and much longer if she chooses to parent her child. This can be a time of great joy as well as emotional stress. To help prepare the teen who opts to keep her child, ask her to discuss all the positive things she associates with motherhood and those she finds disagreeable. (Example: the chance to have an influence on a young life versus morning sickness and dirty diapers.)

To encourage a forward-looking viewpoint, ask the teen to imagine what her child will need and be like in the years to come. It's not hard to think of the needs of a baby, but what does she want for the child in five years? Ten years? Eighteen years? Again, help the young mother set specific goals that might change, yet allow her to develop skills for planning for the future.

Help the teen build her own network of support. This is a group of people on whom she can call for various needs and perhaps to whom she can give in return. Some of the ways they might help include taking her to childbirth class, providing legal or medical help, offering child care while she works or goes to school, supplying clothes and baby items.

Now also is the time to make a budget. Your role as counselor can be pivotal in helping the mother adjust to the discipline of budgeting.

Marriage—Today there is far less social pressure for a "shotgun" wedding. Statistics show that in our divorce-prone society, the vast majority of teen marriages fail when linked to pregnancy before the wedding. Nevertheless, this option needs to be discussed.

Ask the girl to assess her current relationship with the father of the child. Chances are there have been plenty of romantic tinglings, but is there love and commitment as well? Some questions to consider:

1. Is sex the focal point of your relationship, or do you share other interests such as hobbies and favorite subjects?

2. If you were not pregnant, would you still consider the young man your preference for a lifelong mate?

3. Do you agree on the basics of a life together—views about religion, work, childrearing, taking out the garbage, and picking up dirty socks?

4. Do you have the same commitment to rearing this child?

5. Can you accept one another's faults?

Marriage is a partnership. These questions must be addressed to the father of the child as well as to the mother. Be sure both parties have realistic views of marriage. Wedded bliss can sound glamorous, but teens need to face the daily reality of married life. Good marriages can result from teen pregnancies, but they require discipline and hard work.

Adoption—In recent years, this option has become less popular as stigma decreases toward unmarried mothers. Nevertheless, this option deserves careful consideration.

Giving a child for adoption is an act of love that requires maturity on the part of the teen mother in order to anticipate the future needs of her child and accept the fact that others may be better able to meet those needs.

Today, there are many couples who want to be adoptive parents. Some of these couples are Christians who can provide a stable environment, assure the child's schooling and future, as well as provide spiritual nurture.

Laws in many states allow a mother substantial input in selecting adoptive parents. Options may be available that allow contact with the child to be maintained, perhaps through a social service agency. A teen who elects adoption can take practical steps to build a good life for her youngster.

Adoption may be accompanied by its own kind of pain. The mother may go through a grieving process similar to what happens when a child dies. This is a natural reaction which time and supportive counsel will help resolve. The mother will feel reassured knowing her child is in good hands. Although she will never forget her child, the teen mother will be in a position to finish her education and establish direction for her life.

Make Room For Daddy

Male reactions to pregnancy run a full spectrum. Some boys break off the relationship and stop seeing the girl immediately. Other young men want to do the "right thing" by the mother so long as they aren't tied down. Still other boys may demand total control of the situation.

Experts are just beginning to explore the role of fathers as related to teen pregnancy. (See chapter seven for the legal rights of unmarried fathers.) Often these young men are frightened and may appear defiant because, suddenly, they are involved in a situation beyond their control. Reactions vary—they may attempt to shirk responsibility, blame the female, avoid her, or they may feel shunned by the expectant teen and/or her family.

When counseling teen fathers, become familiar with the laws of your state that apply. An attorney, judge, high school counselor, or social service worker can help you.

Begin by helping the father understand the seriousness of the situation and, at the same time, informing him of available help. It is likely he'll need help in long-term planning and goal setting.

Encourage ongoing involvement with the mother and the child if possible. It is important to help him work through his feelings of responsibility and guilt for the circumstances.

Just as for the pregnant teen, help this young man realize his need to purify his lifestyle. The fact that he has been sexually active does not have to continue as a pattern of behavior. The reality of fresh starts is central to the Christian faith. This crisis can have a positive effect on his values and actions.

Crisis pregnancy usually precipitates a turning point in a teen relationship. When great bitterness exists and the father declines to share the experience, it may be wiser to let him waive all rights so the mother will have no complications in making her decision—provided she understands that such freedom could mean loss of financial support.

Handbook for Pregnant Teens suggests these questions as a means of defining the woman's relationship with the father:

1. Would you want the relationship to be different in any other way?
2. How could it be improved?
3. Has it changed since you became pregnant?

4. What kind of relationship do you want the baby and father to have?

5. If you keep the baby but do not marry, what would you want the child to know about the father? [3]

The Grandparents' Perspective

Grandparents, too, can run the full spectrum of emotions. The initial response usually is shock at the sudden transition to being grandparents. There is also the shock that their daughter is being thrust into an adult situation by bearing their grandchild out of the usual sequence of events. At times, the families of the teen mother and father know each other. As a counselor, you will need to monitor this situation—it can be productive, or it can lead to great bitterness.

Expect things to fluctuate. Relationships may be severely tried. Your goal as counselor is not to make all things right, but rather to help families see the broader picture and work for what is best for all concerned. Seek for everyone to face the pregnancy honestly and put away side issues.

A major challenge is the teen mother's needs to now be treated more like an adult. This may be very difficult to accept. She may want to revert to the familiar roles of childhood. Her parents, believing her to have made a major mistake, may insist that she follow their wishes. The argument may be especially strong if they provide financial support. Nevertheless, it is crucial to the ultimate well-being of all that the young mother learn to stand more on her own. The counselor's role can help ease this transition. Begin by suggesting smaller decisions that the mother could make. This will pave the way for a greater sense of responsibility.

After the initial shock, teen pregnancy can bring a family closer together. Mothers who were unable to discuss sex with their daughters may now find common ground in talking about the natural bodily changes of pregnancy. This can bring a new and vital dimension to their relationship.

Grandparents have rights and feelings, too. Individual circumstances will determine the degree to which they should be involved. If the teen mother continues to live under their roof, you probably will see them on a regular basis as you counsel the teen. In such a case, parents must have input to set guidelines for dating, schoolwork, and helping around the house.

Teen mothers must not assume they have built-in baby-sitters. Initially, it may help if the teen mother and her parents draw up a contract of what each party will do to support the other. In time, as people adjust to the reality of the pregnancy, this may be set aside when each side has proven good faith.

Counseling the Teen Who Is Not Pregnant

About 40 percent of women who visit pregnancy centers are not pregnant. When a urine test confirms this, they usually react with great relief. And though their immediate fear has been answered, a basic problem—their life-style—remains to be addressed.

You will find several categories of these women:

1. Young women with relatively few sexual experiences generally are in the under-15 age group. Counseling often reveals that they value sexual involvement as a way to escape problems such as loneliness, desire for popularity, or fear of losing a boyfriend.

2. Teen women who have been sexually involved for one or two years often know about contraceptives but fail to use them properly or at all. They still are uncomfortable with sexual relations. They justify the act when it is spontaneous or "natural" but hesitate to plan for it ahead of time. Many teens at this stage rely on inaccurate "folk wisdom" for prevention of pregnancy. Teens who are not ready for the total realm of adulthood will resist contraceptives, because this signals a great step into the uncertainties of adulthood.

3. Women who accept sexual activity as part of their life-style tend to be in their late teens and twenties. Some are divorced or trapped in unhappy marriages. These women have strong rationales for extramarital sex and may, at first, feel little guilt. But under the surface, many of them are using sex as a "quick fix" to fill a void in life.

Individual responses will vary according to situations, but Scripture's relevancy in diverse settings is a strong indicator of its truth. The Christian Action Council recommends approaches for helping the client evaluate her sexual activity.

In terms of relationships with her boyfriend, sexual relations outside of marriage are destructive. The effect is the opposite of what God intends. It does not draw two people together in a bond of total commitment in which the most expressive means

71

of communication occurs. Instead, sex becomes a means unto itself—a substitute for communication. Sex before commitment thwarts love. Grasping and taking replace the desire to give and share. Too easily, sex becomes the dominant force in a relationship. Is your client feeling this way? These questions will help her identify her feelings:

• How do you feel now that your pregnancy test is negative?
• How might you have felt if your were pregnant?
• How would your boyfriend react if you were pregnant?
• How will this close call affect your relationship?
• How do you feel about being sexually active?
• Who initiates sex in the relationship?
• Do you feel pressured into having sexual relations? If so, to what extent?
• On a scale of 1 to 10 (10 being most comfortable), how do you feel about your overall relationship? About its sexual dimension?

There are several excellent books about sexuality written from a Christian perspective. (See the bibliography for some suggestions). They show that sexual relations, in the proper context, are not dirty or pornographic. Rather, they are created by God for our use and enjoyment. But like food, exercise, or a paycheck, they can be misused, causing harm. As a counselor, you may find these guides to be of special value in discussing an important but sometimes uncomfortable subject.

Having gone through a crisis scare, a young woman in this situation may feel especially vulnerable and angry at herself or her boyfriend. She may feel "used" or "dirty." Consider challenging this woman with a lifestyle that includes secondary virginity. Secondary virginity acknowledges the past sin but offers a fresh start. It's a new commitment on her part. Not that the past will be forgotten, but the grace that is offered through faith in the Lord Jesus Christ, allows Christians to "start over" (I Cor. 6:9-11). Counsel and supportive Christian friends can help her maintain that commitment.

Role Models—An Important Resource

In counseling, it's important to avoid a preachy tone. Show (don't tell) your concern for the people involved in a crisis pregnancy. Also, make as much use as you can of role models. Your clients will respect the words of someone with whom they can identify. In many communities, there are people who have taken the various options—marriage, single parenting, adoption. There are support groups that discuss the unpublicized, negative aspects of abortion. This helps women cope with their personal encounters with abortion. The viewpoints of women who have experienced unwed pregnancy—as well as those of a compassionate counselor—can be of great help to women who now must face the problem.

CHAPTER FIVE

AWARENESS — SO YOU WANT TO GET INVOLVED

TEEN PREGNANCY IS FAR MORE WIDESPREAD TODAY THAN IT was in some past generations, but it still carries an aura of "scandal." The topic of sex invariably leads to gossip, speculation, and fear—even among mature Christians. These dynamics are some of the most destructive forces that can occur within a body of believers. And they are unfair to the individuals who are caught up in the problem. If both the boy and girl (or their families) belong to the same church, this problem can prove divisive for the entire congregation.

Teen pregnancy is a high-pressure problem with many facets. It involves a private sin (sex outside of marriage) with very public consequences. It has physical, emotional, and financial implications. It affects at least three generations of people: teen parents, child, and grandparents.

People learn of the problem through various means. One is the grapevine. Even in a large church, this type of news spreads quickly. What can you do to help, especially if members of the family might come to you for advice?

1. As you work with the family, break the problem into specific components. These would include health care and insurance; attitudes on abortion/adoption/marriage, and single parenting; overall counseling, etc.

2. Convey a clear message to the family and to the church at large: In our fallen world, we expect problems to happen. Of course, the free will of these people led to this problem—but God's grace is designed to forgive and help all those who repent and turn to Him. He's an expert at redeeming "hopeless" situations and working them out for good. A positive, pragmatic approach that does not whitewash sin but also doesn't reject the sinners will serve everyone best.

3. Encourage the family to stay in touch with you. In many cases, they may want to withdraw from the church out of a sense of shame. Remind them that the church is a place that is

designed for treating the real-world hurts that people face. There is no indignity in admitting our needs. Because it is so easy for people to drift away out of embarrassment, you may want to assign someone to stay in particularly close touch with the family. This person should be a mature Christian, possibly a lay leader.

4. If public acknowledgment and confession of sin is practiced in your church, encourage the expectant teen mother and father (if he is also a member of your church) to observe this act of repentance. These young people should not be forced to do this; they must be willing. But you can help them understand the value of such an act. Do all you can to gain the support of the teens and their parents. Point out that the pregnancy cannot easily be kept secret and that there is much benefit in being open and honest before others within the church about our sins. This, of course, will be much easier if this principle has been practiced consistently by other people in the church.

When a teen pregnancy crisis occurs in your church, you will want to take steps to make the congregation aware of how they can show their love and concern for those involved. Even without the crisis occurring in your congregation, your may want to inform people about the frequency and pervasiveness of this problem. Here are some suggestions for meetings you can hold for people within your church: the general congregation, the teens, and parents of teens.

MEETING NO. 1: FOR THE CHURCH

Title: "The Bundle on Our Doorstep"
Objective: To provide for a church-wide discussion of the issue of teenage pregnancy—but not a review of the specific situation.
Time: 1 1/2 to 2 hours

Introduction (five minutes):
(Suggested opening remarks for the leader.)

In generations past, if a young woman became pregnant outside of marriage, she would hide in shame. Soon after delivering her child she might leave the infant—usually in a basket—at the door of a church or a family she trusted, in the hope that they would raise her baby. In some cases, she might scribble a farewell note to the child. Then she would most likely disappear, never to be heard from again. The people who opened the door the next morning faced the challenge: How do we take care of the child?

Today that challenge has increased. An even larger problem has landed on the doorstep of churches like ours. Teen pregnancy is a far more widespread problem. Why? Because premarital sexual activity is so common. And it hits very close to home. According a 1987 survey commissioned by the Josh McDowell Ministry, by age 18, 65 percent of those young people identified as actively participating in evangelical churches had engaged in fondling breasts or genitals; 43 percent had experienced sexual intercourse. [1]

Not only is the problem more common, but its very nature has changed. Today's young mother is not a stranger who arrives and disappears in the night. Very often we know who she is; she may be a member of our own congregation. We see her throughout her pregnancy. We have the opportunity to care for her as well as the baby she is carrying. For this we should be grateful.

Before, that infant in a basket was in danger of exposure until someone opened the door. Today, abortion is legal and popular. An estimated 1.5 million abortions are performed in the U.S. every year—one every 21 seconds. [2] The child's life is in greatest danger before he or she is born. And even after birth, there are physical, emotional, and financial challenges to a single-parent family.

The problem has grown to include many vital social issues. And we must never forget that at the heart of this problem—like all issues facing the church—are individuals in need: a teen mother, her boyfriend, their child, and the grandparents. We are called to serve these people. And we have several avenues open. But to begin, let's hear first-hand from a teen mother as she tells us what she's been going through.

Testimony of Teen Mother (10 minutes):

Ideally, the teen mother should be from outside the church, referred by a social worker or Christian agency. Having gone through the experience, many women are willing to talk about it to groups who want to help.

The woman should have delivered her child already and be established in a stable life-style. She need not be a Christian.

The purpose here is not to analyze her, not to blame her for her situation, and not for her to blame Christians for lack of help. Rather, the goal is to get a first-hand report of what the problem is like and to put a "human face" on the statistics.

She could talk about practical considerations—how she feeds her new family, job opportunities, etc. And she can discuss emotional needs—feeling lonely, tired, and how she stays in touch with friends.

The Larger Picture (10 minutes):
Thank the teen mother for sharing.

Discuss with the group ways your church could have been (or was) involved with this young mother (and others like her) during her pregnancy and ways they now could reach out to her and her child.

Then explain that the real issue involved here is the sanctity and dignity of each human life. Teen mothers feel victimized. Infants are at risk of illness, inadequate care; some infants are at risk of abortion. Link the problem of teen pregnancy to euthanasia, infanticide, condemnation of the handicapped and elderly, and other threats to the sanctity of life.

Motivation for Involvement (30 minutes): (Optional)
Read or hand out excerpts from a book or show a film to inform members of your church about sanctity of life issues. Select a resource that demonstrates why Christians should take a stand, how they can get involved, and how they are able to make a difference. (See the bibliography for suggestions.) The group could discuss the material or roleplay incidents based on the information that was presented.

Raise Two Options (15 minutes):
The problem is serious. As Christians, we need to take a stand. Two avenues are open to us now:

1. Support local, currently existing groups. See what service your community already offers. Birthright, Maternity Homes, Crisis Pregnancy Centers, United Way, and some government agencies address various aspects of the problem. You can urge people to volunteer their time at such places. You also can urge your church to support such works financially as a local missions project.

2. Open your own ministry. If community services are inade-

quate, consider beginning a work. You might want to affiliate with a nationwide network such as the Christian Action Council. Or you might want to share duties with another church/organization.

The following are practical activities that you could begin to undertake:

• Establish a 24-hour crisis hotline. Rotate telephone service linked to the homes of volunteers.

• Provide shelter (in the church or homes of volunteers) to women whose parents or boyfriends have kicked them out. Check local regulations for housing women younger than age 18.

• Collect clothes for pregnant women.

• Arrange transportation to medical appointments or jobs.

• Fund scholarships for teen mothers who want to finish high school.

• Proclaim the pro-life position. Consider writing letters to newspapers and government officials or talk to officials of institutions where abortions are performed, etc. Some may prefer a more public protest at local places where abortions are performed. Such actions must obey laws and avoid violence or destruction of property. Verbal and physical harassment is unacceptable. Protest should be dignified and orderly. Remember: you are not only protesting abortion, you are representing the Christian community. Firmness and love are equally important.

Small Group Discussion (20 minutes):

Set up "information booths" at various places in fellowship hall and staff them with resource people who can provide materials and answer questions. Encourage congregation to stop by each of the booths to talk over ideas, have specific questions answered. Booths could include:

• A teen mother and a social worker who give first-person accounts and local statistics.

• Representatives of community agencies that address the problem.

• Lay church leaders who can discuss the issues scripturally.

Questions from the Floor (15 minutes):

This could be in the style of a town meeting. The people by now have an overview of the issues and should be primed to suggest responses and proposals.

Air various differences; feel the "pulse" of the congregation. You could take motions from the floor or begin to draft proposals on how the church can address this issue.

MEETING NO. 2: FOR THE TEENAGERS

Title: "Teen Pregnancy and You"
Objective: To provide the church teenagers with a safe forum to ask questions, be instructed on the meaning and practice of forgiveness, and emphasize the gravity of the problem.
Time: About one hour

It is important to realize that a single meeting with the teens in your church will not prepare them to meet the sexual pressures of today's world. The most you can hope to do in one session is help your young people respond in a Christian manner to the pregnancy of one of their peers and to get talking constructively about the issue of crisis pregnancy.

It is strongly recommended that you help your church institute a thorough sex education series that emphasizes abstinence. Suggestions for how to launch such a program are presented in the plan for "Meeting No. 3: For Parents Concerned about Prevention."

Introduction (five minutes):

If the teens were not present when you spoke to the whole church about the teen pregnancy in the congregation, share the information as outlined at the beginning of this chapter. Otherwise, just review it briefly.

Explain that the purpose of this session together is to answer any questions the teens may have, review the meaning and practice of forgiveness, and discuss the matter of teen pregnancy. In this regard you will want to guide the discussions away from the specific situation as soon as any necessary information has been provided.

The Importance of Forgiveness (15 minutes):

It would be ideal if you could invite an adult woman who bore a child out of wedlock to share her experience as a teenage mother, particularly emphasizing the impact of those who did and did not accept her. This, however, need not be a person from your church. Such a person could be contacted through organizations such as Birthright, Maternity Homes, or Crisis Pregnancy Centers. If the person is known to the teenagers, be sure that the no one will be embarrassed or harmed by the discussion.

The biblical importance of forgiveness can be reviewed in David's experience (II Sam. 11—12, Ps. 51), the woman taken in adultery (John 8:1-11), and the requirement to forgive (Matt. 18:21-35).

Encourage the young people to share experiences (probably from earlier childhood) when they were ostracized because of what others said about them—true or not.

Attitudes toward Teen Pregnancy (15 minutes):

Get the kids thinking about their attitudes toward teen pregnancy. You don't want to interrogate them personally or "snoop" on their friends. Keep questions open-ended and general.

Here are some questions to get you going:
• Do kids you know talk a lot about pregnancy?
• What do kids think of sex before or outside of marriage?
• Without giving names, how many people do you know who are sleeping together? Has this number gone up or down over the past few years?
• At what age do teens become sexually active?
• At what stage in a relationship does sexual activity begin?
• Who initiates it? Why?
• What do guys expect out of sex? What do girls expect? (Males and females should answer separately)
• What do teens who sleep together know about birth control? Do they use it? Each time? According to directions? If they don't use it, why not?
• Let's talk about each option. What do you think about: marriage? adoption? single parenting? abortion?
• What do you think the guy's role should be when his girlfriend gets pregnant? Does he have special responsibilities? Does he have any rights or a say in what goes on?

The Tragedy of Abortion (15 minutes):

Using the content of chapters one, two, and six from this book, guide a discussion on the nature and tragedy of abortion

81

today.

Begin by asking the group how many know someone who has had an abortion. Ask for volunteers to share (*without revealing names or identifiable facts*). Ask questions such as:
• Why did she choose to have an abortion?
• How do you think the experience affected her?
• Do you think she would have another abortion? Why?
• What other options might she have reasonably chosen?

You will need to be careful in leading this portion of the session if the girl in your church hasn't yet made her decision to carry the baby to term. Also, there may be other women in the church (even the youth group) who have already had abortions. It is very important to maintain the balance between God's preventative standards and His forgiveness. We are all sinners and have no business "sinner-bashing"—stirring negative group sentiment against any category of sinners or whipping up guilt in people whom God has forgiven.

Helpful Responses (10 minutes):

Allow time to invite the group's input for how they might reach out to pregnant teens—volunteering with such organizations as Birthright, Maternity Homes, and Crisis Pregnancy Centers, committing themselves to reach out in friendship, speaking up in discussions at school for abstinence, etc.

MEETING NO. 3: FOR PARENTS CONCERNED ABOUT PREVENTION

Title: "How to Encourage Sexual Abstinence Before Marriage"
Objective: To allow parents to review some of the available sex education materials that promote abstinence. To enlist their support for launching such a program in your church.
Time: About 90 minutes.
Special, Advance Preparation Required: See the second step, "Possible Options."

Introduction: (15 minutes)
As necessary, review the problem:
• Briefly review statistics regarding the sexual activity of teens. (You may want to refer to the first chapter of this book and to the survey commissioned by the Josh McDowell Ministry that is

mentioned on page 77 of this chapter.)
• An estimated 1.5 million abortions are performed in the U.S. every year—one every 21 seconds. [3]
• Briefly mention any teenage pregnancies that have occurred within the congregation. Focus on the problem, not the individuals who were involved.

The Bible teaches that sexual relations are created by God and ordained for human pleasure and procreation. But like all things in this world, specific rules apply for our well-being. An understanding of these principles is essential for a teenager to become a successful, independent, and mature adult.

It's never been easy for parents to discuss sex with their children. That's especially true today, because of the tremendous changes in social values that have occurred in recent years. Your children are literally living in a different world than the one in which you grew up.

Years ago, sex was hushed up, never discussed between parents and children or in society at large. Information came from friends, "on the street" or by experimentation. Think back: how much did your parents talk with you? Where did you acquire your sexual information?

Today the schools are trying to fill the vacuum, but too often their efforts to be "value neutral" appear to give permission, if not encouragement, for sexual experimentation. What can we do?

Possible Options (50 minutes):

A number of organizations have developed sex education materials which encourage teenagers to say "no" to premarital sex. Some are designed for use in public schools while others are better suited for use in churches. Here are some of the programs that promote teen sexual abstinence:

The Foundation for the Family, Inc.
P.O. Box 389155
Cincinnati, OH 45238

Search Institute
122 West Franklin Ave., Suite 215
Minneapolis, MN 55404

Sex Respect
Respect, Inc.
347 S. Center
Bradley, IL 60915

Teen-Aid, Inc.
North 1330 Calispel
Spokane, WA 99201

Teen Star
8514 Bradmore Dr.
Bethesda, MD 20817

Why Wait?
Box 1000
Dallas, TX 75221

Before the session, order samples and/or promotional information from the above groups and any materials available through your church denomination. Initially review them with your church's youth leadership or other appropriate persons, and bring the three top curricula for the parents' inspection and final selection.

Group Evaluation and Selection (25 minutes):
When evaluating which curriculum would be best for your church, here are a few questions that you might encourage the parents to ask:

• Does this material present a biblically positive view of sex, in contrast to a perspective that sees it as merely necessary or even slightly dirty?
• Does it adequately emphasize the importance of abstinence before marriage, or is this only presented as "one of the options"?
• Does the program have a way to include the parents, facilitating and helping them to maintain a role in their child's sex education?
• Does this program speak accurately about current teenage sexual trends and attitudes? On what is this authority based? (Nothing is worse than for a program to be obviously out of date

on a subject like this.)

• Does this program explain in clear and convincing ways the incremental steps that a teenager needs to take to avoid sexual involvement? Or does it imply that early dating and intimate behavior can be managed while saying "no" at the last minute to premarital intercourse?

• What are the positive ways it suggests for young people to deal with their sexual tension?

• Is the curriculum designed in such a way that *your* teachers can present it effectively? Or does it beg for some kind of an "expert" who is not available in your church?

• What do other churches that have used this material have to say about it? (A few phone calls can be very worthwhile. Ask the publisher for names and numbers.)

Conclude the meeting by arriving at a decision or a final recommendation to be taken back to your curriculum committee.

CHAPTER SIX

ABORTION — NOT A CHOICE FOR CHRISTIANS

"IT IS EASY FOR CHRISTIANS TO BE PRO-LIFE . . . UNTIL THEIR daughter gets pregnant." I heard that statement more than a year ago, and the passing of time has not diminished my surprise and hurt that someone could say it. I had hoped the view was an isolated one. Unfortunately, interviews with teen mothers, social workers, pastors, and counselors show that it is an all-too-common response in our Christian world.

You can see how ethics can easily slip. Most Christians have a general sense that life is sacred, but there are few occasions to put that belief to the test. When pregnancy engulfs a family, however, general concepts can be overwhelmed by stress. There is great pressure to "solve the problem and get on with life." Few people sense the irony in that statement.

Of course, many Christians boldly defend life, even when doing so is inconvenient, expensive, and emotionally wrenching. But sometimes even these people are unable to articulate just why they take such a stand. Or they're searching for a foundation of truth to help them cope with the particulars of their own situation.

To establish a firm foundation for what we as Christians think about abortion, let's consider some specific questions.

What Is Abortion?

The dictionary defines abortion as "the expulsion or removal of an embryo or fetus from the womb at a stage of pregnancy when it is incapable of independent survival."[1] Spontaneous abortions or "miscarriages" occur in many pregnancies. Induced abortion is another matter. Throughout much of American history, this procedure was condemned by physicians, jurists, and leaders of social action movements. A sweeping change occurred in January 1973.

Resulting in millions of abortions, the decision by the United States Supreme Court on *Roe vs. Wade* determined:

• Abortion is legal for any reason in the first three months of pregnancy if a licensed physician performs the procedure.

• During the middle third of pregnancy, abortion is legal for any reason, but states individually may pass laws to protect the health of the mother. (This recognizes the increased risk of medical complication with abortions at later stages of pregnancy.)

• During the last third of pregnancy, when many children could survive outside the womb, abortion still is legal if the mother and her doctor decide it is necessary for the woman's life and health. In analyzing this ruling, Curt Young of the Christian Action Council states, "The health exception is defined so broadly as to permit abortion for any reason." [2]

The key issue is whether abortion takes a human life or, as many advocates of abortion claim, is merely the removal of tissue that has the *potential* for human life. The definitions of certain words are important in understanding this critical issue.

Embryo is the term that refers to the early stages of development. In humans, it generally refers to the first trimester (three months) of life. After that, the individual usually is called a *fetus*. After birth, the individual is called an infant, a baby, a toddler, a child, an adolescent, and so on, all the way to senior citizen. But all of these terms *describe* stages of development. There is no point after conception when the life "becomes" human. It has been so from the start.

This claim cannot be made for either the egg or the sperm prior to their union. There is nothing viably human or potentially human in either of them alone. As it has been aptly said, the only situation in which we can rightly claim the *potential for human life* is when 200 million eager sperm are chasing an egg in a fallopian tube. But once the sperm and egg have joined, human life has begun.

Of course, throughout the person's development his or her appearance changes greatly, but from conception throughout all of life, only three material things are added to the ongoing development of that person: food, oxygen, and a suitable environment. There is no point when something else is infused into the being to change its nature, and there is no point when any one of those three supports can be withdrawn.

Some people have suggested that "viability" is the standard for defining when human life begins. But this vague term has a variety of meanings. In *Roe vs. Wade*, the Supreme Court definition of viability can be summarized as "capable of independent existence."

But subsequent scientific developments show how inadequate and subjective this definition is. Children who were "not viable" (able to live independent of the mother) when abortion was legalized now can be saved through routine medical care. In fact, viability is not so much a description of the child's development as it is a description of the state of our scientific art to offer the three supports for all life: food, oxygen, and a suitable environment.

Curt Young points out that before the Supreme Court legalized it, abortion was defined as "the expulsion of a fetus from the womb before it is viable"—independent of the mother. To destroy a *viable* fetus or newborn child was to commit infanticide, "the murder of a baby." Medical advances mean that viability is coming earlier in many pregnancies, in some cases as early as five months. But since it is legal to have an abortion at any time in pregnancy, viable infants now are being killed.

In fact, in some instances we must even deal with "failed" procedures in which the aborted child is delivered alive and then killed.

But children are becoming increasingly at risk after birth, too. In the 1982 Indiana case of "Infant Doe," a Down's syndrome baby was allowed to starve to death. The boy was born with a detached esophagus, which routine surgery could have corrected. Unable to take food through the mouth, he was denied tube feedings and surgical treatment.

His parents, the doctor, and the courts agreed to let this boy starve to death, in spite of the fact that nearly a dozen families offered to adopt him. The *Chicago Tribune* commented. "It is a measure of abortion's effect on our thinking that in at least one state it is now permissible to do to a deformed, retarded infant what would be illegal if done to a dog or cat." [3]

"Quickening" has also been proposed as the definition of when human life begins. It refers to the mother's perception of active life within her body. But again, the reference here is not the fetus, but the mother's subjective ability to feel. Nothing qualitative has changed in the baby. He or she has just reached a certain point of weight and strength when movements become apparent to the mother.

What Does Man Say?

How have we reached this state of affairs where we are calling human beings "fetal tissue" because they are not "viable" (or even if they are) and thereby excusing their destruction? Has this been a common understanding throughout history? Are pro-life people trying to insist on some new or narrowly defined religious ethic?

Michael J. Gorman has traced the dynamics among pagan, Jewish, and Christian thinking in his book, *Abortion and the Early Church*. His scholarly analysis gives thorough treatment to this complex subject. For the purpose of summary, it is safe to say pagan societies often viewed life as utilitarian and expendable. And in application of the adage, "might makes right," those who were weakest suffered most. [4]

Ancient Greece and Rome

The status of unborn children was variable; their rights usually were overshadowed by other concerns. For example, ancient Greeks gave first consideration to the needs of the state. Although some philosophers, including Plato, considered the fetus to be a living being, the collective needs of society were more important than the personal needs of individuals.

When it came to a choice, the state's needs prevailed, whether it meant the death of a fetus or of someone already born. Unwanted infants were "exposed"—abandoned to death via starvation, animal attack, or exposure. At various times in Greek history, female and handicapped infants were especially vulnerable; aged and disabled adults suffered much the same fate.

The general thinking was that only those who could contribute meaningfully to the state deserved its full protection. In this context, abortion became an attractive option, whether people wished to limit family size, retain a youthful figure, or hide the consequence of illicit sexual relations.

Ancient Rome had a more consistent view of the fetus. The fetus was considered part of the mother's viscera—not independently human. But humans themselves had varying rights. Throughout much of its history, Rome gave primacy to the father—who could force his wife (and servants) to have an abortion, or demand punishment for abortions performed without his consent. Abortion and exposure were common occurrences, seemingly compatible with the popular mindset that lauded gladiator fights and executions as public entertainment.

The Judaeo-Christian Tradition

Today, it's easy to oversimplify our Judaeo-Christian heritage. Judaism and Christianity differ in significant respects, and each has faced internal divisions.

But when contrasted with the values of other societies, Judeo-Christian ethics do stand apart and therefore can be viewed together. This is especially true of valuing human life, both born and unborn. In its classic form, the Judaeo-Christian tradition alone gives eternal value to each individual. This is not based on the person's contribution to society but because he or she is made in the image of God.

Jewish law and tradition developed over a period of at least 1,500 years. The Hebrew Bible and the writings of the rabbis covered the most minute facets of human life. These writings contain vigorous debate about how to apply divine principles in daily life. Yet throughout this complex, comprehensive work, there is virtually no reference to abortion by choice. Why? Gorman explains: "It was a given of Jewish thought and life that abortion, like exposure, was unacceptable."[5] Opinions differed within Judaism about when a fetus received a human soul and what punishment was appropriate for accidental abortion. But no Jewish leader ever considered abortion unless the mother's life was in grave danger. (Provision was even made for accepting the children of Jewish mothers who were raped by non-Jews.)

The Jewish nation evidently agreed with their leaders. Throughout ancient Jewish writings, there is a marked absence of legal records involving lawsuits for abortion by choice or official decrees to regulate abortion. Had these existed, they might indicate the subject was a concern to society. Instead, Jews regarded pregnancy in terms of: "first, the duty and desire to populate the earth and ensure both Jewish survival and the divine presence; second, a deep sense of the sanctity of life as God's creation, a respect extending in various ways to life in all its manifestations and stages; and, finally, a profound horror of blood and bloodshed."[6]

Christianity, as it grew, broke from Judaism in several key respects. But it retained and built upon the fundamental Jewish regard for human life. As the early church was defining its standards, it confronted the question of abortion directly and took a clear stand. *The Didache*, an early church manual, declared: "Thou shalt not murder a child by abortion/destruction."[7]

In A.D. 197, Tertullian wrote, "In our case, murder being once for all forbidden, we may not destroy even the fetus in the womb, while as yet the human being derives blood from other parts of the body for its sustenance. To hinder a birth is merely a speedier man-killing; nor does it matter whether you take away a life that is born, or destroy one that is coming to the birth."[8]

There are very few records of abortion on demand among the ancient Jews. Early Christians, however, were not a distinct ethnic or geographic group. Their numbers were increasing amid persecutions of varying intensity. Abortions did occur within the early church. But rather than accommodate the practice, early Christian leaders stood firm and emphasized that abortion was murder, even when such a position meant the condemnation of wealthy, powerful families within the young church.

Gorman notes that Hippolytus wrote this rebuke not long after Tertullian's warning: "Women, reputed believers, began to resort to drugs for producing sterility, and to gird themselves round, so to expel what was being conceived on account of their not wishing to have a child either by a slave or any paltry fellow, for the sake of their family and excessive wealth. Behold, into how great impiety that lawless one has proceeded, by inculcating adultery and murder at the same time!"[9]

The problem of crisis pregnancy did not go away, but the church maintained its clear position. Basil of Caesarea, a leader of the Eastern church, reviewed the problem in A.D. 374. Note that he rejects hair-splitting about when human life begins during fetal development.

She who has deliberately destroyed a fetus has to pay the penalty of murder. And there is no exact inquiry among us as to whether the fetus was formed or unformed. For, here it is not only the child to be born that is vindicated, but also the woman herself who made an attempt against her own life, because usually the women die in such attempts. Furthermore, added to this is the destruction of the embryo, another murder, at least according to the intention of those who dare these things.[10]

Curt Young of the Christian Action Council notes that the church has been divided over a number of fundamental issues in its nearly 2,000 years of history. But at no time—even the traumatic schism of 1054 and the Protestant Reformation of 1517 —has the value of human life undergone debate. Reformer John Calvin declared that "the fetus, though enclosed in the womb of its mother, is already a human being and it is a most monstrous crime to rob it of the life which it has not yet begun to enjoy. If it seems more horrible to kill a man in his own house than in a field, because a man's house is his place of most secure refuge, it ought surely to be deemed more atrocious to destroy a fetus in the womb before it has come to light." [11]

Modern Aberrations

The writings of Francis Schaeffer make it clear that a battle continually rages over the direction a society will take. In the Bible, God has given a clear and absolute standard. Part of that standard defines all human life as sacred. That standard is hateful to Satan and contrary to our fallen nature.

Not surprisingly, then, it is under constant attack. The type of attack varies. It may come through channels of law, the popular arts, science, philosophy, or economics. But its purpose never changes: to undermine what God has decreed (which also happens to be what is best for us) on this earth and to prevent our eternal reconciliation with Him through Christ.

Against this attack, we have God's law to guide our conduct and the promise of divine help to carry out God's will. But it's up to us to use these resources: God will not force our hand. Unless we identify and hold fast to the values we cherish, they will be eroded and replaced by what we abhor.

Schaeffer's book, *The Great Evangelical Disaster*, charts the remarkable speed with which traditional values have disintegrated in America. He writes that the United States never was a truly Christian nation, but until 60 years ago there was a "Christian consensus" that influenced American society as a whole—especially our attitudes toward marriage and the family.

The challenge in those earlier times was to persuade people that the Bible's straightforward values should be incorporated into everyday life. Today, however, people no longer even see the Bible as a source of specific values.

What belief is replacing the sanctity of life that God spells out in the Bible? The new concept arrives with a beguiling name, "quality of life." It sounds so decent: Every child should be

93

wanted; every life should be worth living. Yet the other side of this idea is quite ominous: An "unworthy" life should not be lived. And the frightening question now becomes, who will decide which life is "worthy"?

But what explains the remarkable consistency that Christians held over the centuries? It lies in the emphasis our faith places upon the individual. Christ died to provide salvation for all people, but the choice to accept His gift falls to each person alone. Each of us has a distinct personality to be valued and protected. We are compelled to explore how the Bible guided ancient Jews and Christians to consider human life sacred from the moment of conception until natural death.

What Does God Say?

Families are important to God. He uses the earthly family as a metaphor to explain eternal truths. Terms such as "Father," "Son," and "my brothers" help convey the sense of a God who is in complete control of the universe yet knows each of us by name.

Families contain the daily drama of life: love, ambition, disappointment. The Bible does not sugar-coat the family, but uses the model of the family to illustrate truths about our relationship with God and one another.

Most important, the Bible shows us that God intervenes when families in crisis turn to Him. For example, Moses' mother could not keep her child, and Mary's baby, soon after birth, was threatened by the brutality of a great king. God doesn't deal in answers that are tentative or the better of two evils. His redemption represents what is truly best for everyone concerned. This extends to defenseless children (Jas. 1:27) and certainly to the weakest people of all, the unborn.

The Bible does not have many parables or teachings that deal overtly with the problem of teenage pregnancy as we know it today. For one thing, in Bible times people usually married *before* they reached sexual maturity. It hasn't been until modern times that marriage was commonly postponed until five to seven years after puberty. For a variety of nutritional and environmental reasons, puberty is occurring earlier while marriage is delayed until after years of education and vocational training, leaving the utterly modern phenomena of five to seven years of "adolescence"—all of this in a society with greatly increased sexual stimulation through the media. But the Bible does illuminate the key principles of conduct that are useful in coping with crisis pregnancies. [12]

1. God alone is the Author of life.

In Genesis 1:26-27 and 5:1-3 the Bible uses parallel wording to describe how Seth reflects the likeness of his father, Adam, just as Adam reflects the likeness of his Creator, God. Also in these early accounts we see that God gave humans dominion over the earth and all the plants and animals. But significantly missing is any mention of our having dominion over human life. God alone is sovereign over human life.

Some of the most intense personal struggles in the Bible involve childbearing. Hagar and Sarah's animosity toward each other (Gen. 16:21), Isaac and Rebekah's desire for a child (Gen. 25:21), Leah and Rachel's conflict (Gen. 29:31; 30:2, 22), and Hannah's desire for a child (I Sam. 1)—all recount how God "opened the womb" and made new life possible. Whatever their differences, everyone looked to God as the Source of all life.

In many other passages, the Old Testament saints acknowledge God as the Source of their life. Psalm 71:6 is a particular illustration of this: "From birth I have relied on you; you brought me forth from my mother's womb." Other passages affirming the same truth can be found in Job 33:4; Psalms 8:4-9; 31:15; 95:6; 100:3; 104:29, 30; 119:73; 127:3.

God's authority over human life is a theme that spans both Old and New Testaments. The translation saying Mary was "with child" uses a figure of speech that was common into this century (over-modest Victorians preferred it to "pregnant," which struck them as being too explicit). But the clear meaning was that the pregnant woman was carrying a *human child*, not the "product of conception" or "reproductive tissue" in today's parlance. And the unique circumstances of Mary's pregnancy vividly demonstrate that God alone is the Creator of life.

When Paul addressed the people of Athens in the middle of the Areopagus, he said, "The God who made the world and everything in it is the Lord of heaven and earth and does not live in temples built by hands. And he is not served by human hands, as if he needed anything, because he himself gives all men life and breath and everything else" (Acts 17:24, 25).

2. The fetus is fully human.

Scripture holds that human life is a continuum, only a part of which takes place on earth.

God has a specific plan for each person, which he occasionally reveals even before that person is born. The relationship between Jacob and Esau was determined prior to their birth (Gen. 25:23; Rom. 9:10-12). The parents of Samson (Judg. 13:3-5), John the Baptist (Luke 1:15), and Jesus (Luke 1:30, 41-44; 2:21) all learned about their offspring before their births—with such details as name, life-style, and type of service.

The Bible treats pregnancy as a natural part of the human experience, which carries on throughout earthly life. Just as the Bible gives specific information about a person before birth, it also shows how the individual personality continues after death. (See the account of Lazarus and the rich man in Luke 16.) In talking about the process of life, the Bible never asks, "When does it all begin?" The Bible is based upon what medical science is still grappling to accept: the fact that life begins at conception.

It may be surprising to know how often the Bible mentions God's active involvement with the fetus. The womb is a frequent point of reference (Ps. 139:13-16). Scripture reveals God working there, weaving, molding, and pouring our lives into shape. This is not a God who is indifferent to our fate; He can count the hairs on our heads.

Why does the Bible emphasize God's work within the womb? One reason is to show His complete sufficiency and supremacy. Life could not begin without Him. To work in this setting reveals God's tender mercy and ultimate mastery in relationship to us. It also shows God's commitment to the weak and helpless, for who is more vulnerable than a pregnant woman and her developing fetus? By caring for their needs, God shows His willingness to provide for us at every juncture of life.

3. We are not to decide another person's "quality of life."

It's not easy to admit weakness. No one enjoys confronting the fact that life is short and full of disappointment. Everyone faces limitations. Moses, for instance, complained about his lack of eloquence, thinking that he was ill-equipped to do the task God had assigned for him to do. But the Lord responded: "Who gave man his mouth? Who makes him deaf or mute? Who gives him sight or makes him blind? Is it not I, the Lord?" (Exod. 4:11).

Yet many people try to deny the existence of our human frailty, often by turning against those who seem weaker, perhaps as an attempt to assert strength.

In many passages the Bible shows how we should support one another and how God will support us. If Moses had been perfect, how could people have seen God's role in their deliverance?

Isaiah points out that we have no right to rebuke God for our earthly condition (Isa. 45:9-11). Each life is sacred and purposeful, despite what we perceive to be shortcomings.

Many books and articles today argue that people who are seriously disabled have the right to end their own lives. On an even more chilling note, other people believe that disabled individuals have a "duty" to die so society is not burdened by the business of caring for "unproductive" members. This was a prime tenet of Nazi doctrine and is cropping up again in arguments favoring euthanasia.

Yet some of the most persuasive messages of human dignity and God's love come from people who are considered "worthless." Can anyone doubt Helen Keller's impact in showing that handicapped people can enjoy "quality of life"? And who would discount the influence of Joni Earickson Tada, who was paralyzed as a teenager but has used her disability to demonstrate God's provision?

As the Great Physician, Jesus came to help the sick. All of us have the disease of sin, but many people refuse to recognize it—and refuse to seek Christ's help for it. People who continue to insist they have no need of Christ, His love, and forgiveness will find themselves permanently denied. So, too, will those who refuse to help people in need. Christ rejected no one who came to Him. In Matthew 25 we see how Jesus identified with the poor and weak. To neglect or abuse them is an assault on Jesus Himself: "Whatever you did not do for one of the least of these, you did not do for me" (Matt. 25:45).

4. God gives a place of honor to children.

Children are uniquely important in God's order for the world. As the Lord's legacy, they provide for the continuation of the human race. Psalm 127:3 reminds us that children "are a heritage from the Lord . . . a reward from him." As helpless creatures, children can bring out expressions of unselfish love in adults; children can establish a relationship that lets us see how

God looks at us.

God's penchant for using the weak to confound and teach the strong appears in the role He assigns children. The example of a child can lead all of us (Matt. 18:1-6). When we become too aware of our own worth or accomplishments, we must recall that there is no place for boasting in the kingdom of God.

Children truly are defenseless. God told the Hebrew people to "Leave your orphans; I will protect their lives. Your widows too can trust in me" (Jer. 49:11). God is deeply concerned about the helpless, and this certainly applies to the child of a crisis pregnancy. In many cases, the birth father will have nothing to do with his girlfriend and child. And in cases where the mother wants an abortion, the child has dire need of an advocate. Concerned citizens must step forward to defend the child's right to live.

What is to happen to children who are "fatherless"—who lack the family structure God has ordained? The Bible is clear: A place must be found for them. The Bible shows that adoption is a viable option. In fact, it's one that all Gentile Christians have experienced personally when they enter God's spiritual family (Eph. 2:19).

As a Gentile, I have no natural right to belong to the household of faith. My ancestors in the British isles were painting themselves blue and talking to trees while the ancient Hebrews were in communion with the true God. Through no merit of my own, I have been grafted onto the "true vine" of faith. Conversely, as Paul explains, Jews who do not believe in their own Messiah have cut themselves off from the root of their faith (Rom. 11:17, 18). But the wonder of Jesus is that He makes room for all, Gentile and Jew, to believe in Him and "abide" in Him, as Jesus explained in John 15.

What Can We Do?

As we saw earlier, the church initially took a clear stand on the value of unborn human life, and it followed this precedent with remarkable consistency until our own generation. Conversely, secular institutions and leaders have wavered throughout the centuries. At various times, they have agreed with the Christian view (although for different reasons), attacked it, and been influenced by it. Today, through such powerful forces as the United States Supreme Court, secular influence aggressively combats traditional Christian thinking.

In calling believers to be salt and light, Jesus expected His followers to live in contrast to the world's values. Tension between Christianity and its surrounding culture was evident from the beginning, but given the fluid and highly charged environment of this present day, our challenge is to hold fast to the central tenets of Christian faith. Prominent among them is the sacred value of human life.

But what can we do? It's one thing to decry the negative drift in our collective values. But the issue jolts into real-world clarity when you face a pregnant teenager. Her problems represent vast connotations for our society. Right now, however, she needs clothes for her changing figure, guidance about her education and career, reassurance for her anxiety. We must start out by helping her. Our efforts will have benefits on a scale more vast than we would think.

Jesus ministered to individuals. It's at this same personal level that you can make a difference. You can help specific young women who are in need. And by doing so, you'll add a bulwark to the wayward drift of our society.

In Fullerton, California, members of the First Evangelical Free Church held a series of meetings to determine what the congregation could do about abortion. Committees for professional care, counseling, practical care (clothing, transportation, housing), and education were established. A four-bedroom house was purchased as a maternity home and church members serve as house parents. In many ways, this kind of direct help is the most essential response.

But there are other options—the creation of counseling centers to reach out to women who are experiencing a crisis pregnancy, public information efforts aimed at informing people of the dangers of abortion and encouraging changes in hospital policies, and involvement and support for good adoption programs.

In the next chapter we will look at some of the resources available for pregnant teens.

CHAPTER SEVEN

RESOURCES FOR SUPPORTING NEW LIFE

S O THE YOUNG MOTHER-TO-BE HAS MADE HER DECISION TO carry her child to term. This is a cause for celebration. As Moses urged, she has chosen life rather than death, and God will bless her for it (Deut. 30). But that doesn't mean all her problems have been solved. This chapter is designed as a resource guide concerning various legal concerns, a general description of adoption procedures, questions often asked about adoption, and agencies and programs to support the single mother. Contact your local authorities for specific help and information needed for individuals you're serving.

It is important to be alert to the attitudes of the women you help. Their feelings will make a tremendous difference in the kind of assistance they require and their own willingness to cooperate with helpers. Some families want to explore every option to make the best decision for all parties. Other families have their minds made up or simply want to let things "drift" with a minimum of personal involvement. Temper your activity to match the needs and desires of the people you're helping. It's fine to expose them to a range of options and even to help them think through decisions, but you must realize that the responsibility and decision-making power is theirs.

When Do People Need Legal Assistance?

Laws related to teen and crisis pregnancies are not fixed in concrete. Regulations may vary widely among states, and individuals may have very different needs.

The goal of this chapter is not to present a systematic analysis of the laws that apply to all situations of unplanned pregnancy. As legal concerns develop, it is essential that you contact experts in your own community for help. This chapter will only take a survey approach, outlining some of the major issues you should be aware of, some of the trends in the response to this problem, and some of the useful resources available at the local level. We will examine the role of law in crisis pregnancy from the viewpoint of the mother, father, grandparents, and third-party helpers. We'll take a look at times when legal considerations need to be addressed and some of the most frequently asked questions that deal with legal issues in pregnancy.

Many aspects of a crisis pregnancy can be handled by concerned individuals, helpful church volunteers, social workers, and doctors. At times, however, it is helpful to involve attorneys and even the police. Of course, every situation differs, but you should monitor instances such as the following for possible involvement of the authorities:

• *Animosity among the parties*—Crisis pregnancy typically brings strong emotions to the forefront. It's best for people to work through their own differences, but sometimes this isn't possible. Resentment and anger may translate into "conspiracies." And if one person feels intimidated or neglected in the decision-making process, the involvement of a lawyer may help assure a more balanced approach. Keep in mind, however, that a lawyer generally represents the interests of one party and doesn't act as a "referee."

• *Physical abuse*—A woman's home environment may be unsafe. If she faces any physical danger whatsoever, the police should be notified. State laws, in fact, may require such reporting, especially in cases involving minors. Short-term "crisis housing" may be required, or she may need shelter for the duration of her pregnancy. Be attentive to situations where the woman is in danger but does not want to leave home. Problems may cool down for the moment, especially if the abuser knows that others are concerned about the woman's well-being. Promises to reform, though, are not always so diligently kept, and the situation could deteriorate again.

• *Alcohol or chemical abuse*—Sometimes the woman's parent or partner has a dependency problem that can aggravate the home situation. This may heighten her need for alternative housing.

In other cases, the mother herself may have a dependency problem with alcohol or other drugs. This can be extremely hazardous for both woman and fetus. Proper care should involve an authentic chemical abuse program such as those that use the steps developed by Alcoholics Anonymous. A "general" counselor may not be sufficient; breaking a chemical dependency usually requires specialized care. If the woman persists in breaking the law and endangering the health of herself and her child, the police may need to be notified. No one wants to see a pregnant woman go to jail, but a mother is not above the law, either. And sometimes a warning from the police can induce a woman to seek the necessary therapy to break such destructive patterns of behavior.

• *Rape/incest*—Pregnancy can result from cases of rape and incest. These events, especially involving a minor, should be reported to the police. There is also a social and ethical responsibility to report this type of incident. Legal counsel may be advisable.

It can be extremely difficult for a woman to "go public" at such a time, but in a noncoercive manner you should encourage her to acknowledge that she has been attacked. This can be the best way to begin the healing process.

It is also critically important for the woman to get the counseling and medical assistance necessary to help put the experience behind her. Tragically, many women feel that they are in some way to blame for such attacks. By working with compassionate experts, the woman can see that she is in fact a victim.

There may be a stressful, lengthy interval (often several years) before the pain of such an event disappears. But the benefits of confronting the problem make the effort worthwhile. Lawyers and police, as dispassionate experts, can help victims go through the process of recovery.

Adoption: Choices and Challenges

Today, adoption usually requires legal counsel. Laws vary considerably among states; also, the concept of adoption itself is changing. The decisions made will have long-term consequence for parents and children. For an excellent discussion of this subject, *A Guide to Adoption* is recommended. Published in 1988 by Focus on the Family, this book was written by Douglas R. Donnelly, an attorney from California.

Fifty years ago, adoptions related to teen pregnancy were fairly informal, especially in rural areas. A girl would become pregnant and, if she did not have a "shotgun" wedding, would be sent to stay with relatives or friends in a distant community. Soon after birth, the child would be processed through a loose network of neighbors, relations, pastors, and doctors. Often, no papers were ever signed. The child simply became part of another family, in some cases living quite close to the birth mother. Such was the case for Ethel Waters, whose autobiography is reviewed in the bibliography of this book. Her mother was 12 years old when Ethel was born. Ethel was reared by her grandmother and aunts; she considered her mother an older sister.

By the end of World War II, however, adoption in the United States was becoming strictly formalized. Neutral third parties, such as social service agencies, handled most cases. Legal papers had to be signed. Information was held in close confidence, with the goal of making a total separation between birth mother and child. Many children grew up never knowing they were adopted. When they did try to locate their birth parents, they ran up against a formidable wall of red tape. Today there are books and support groups that help people from this generation find information about their birth parents.

Adoption today combines elements of both the informal and highly structured approaches used earlier. In many cases, today's methods combine the best components of each. Basically, there are two distinct schools of thought at present. They differ markedly.

• *Agency adoption*—This more conventional approach has been criticized as bureaucratic and impersonal, but reforms are making it more amenable to individual needs. The role of an agency is to serve as intermediary.

Agencies that handle adoption must be reviewed and licensed, usually by the state. As long as they meet established guidelines, agencies, however, may reflect a certain value system. For example, there are agencies with a specific evangelical emphasis.

Agencies provide a host of services such as education for the pregnant teen. They also provide emotional, physical, and legal protection and support. They require certain specific criteria to be met by the people who participate in the adoptive process. As a model, we will describe the approach taken by the Crisis Pregnancy Center where my wife, Lea, works. Contact the agencies in your area to see how they compare.

When a woman elects to carry her child to term, the CPC advises her to take several months to decide if she will parent the child alone or place it for adoption. By the seventh month of pregnancy, this decision should be crystalizing. For the sake of this example, we will assume the mother chooses adoption.

During the eighth and ninth month, Crisis Pregnancy Center staff members discuss what the mother can expect after delivering her baby. These talks include the legal process of adoption, the emotional response and grieving process of this decision, and practical issues, such as whether she wants visitors in the hospital to see the baby.

After the child's birth, on the mother's last day in the hospital, she signs papers to release her child to a foster home (which has been approved by the agency). She still retains all legal rights to the child; however, she does not have the right to decide in which home her child shall be placed.

The child may remain in foster care for up to several months. During this time the mother and, if she agrees, the father may visit the child. Grandparents also may have visiting rights.

If all parties agree that adoption should go forward, there can be a *voluntary signing* away of rights. The child's parents (and if the parents are minors, the grandparents as well) sign a statement, which has legal force, provided by the agency. The signing can take place in the hospital soon after birth or after a period of foster care. Following the signing, all parties have ten working days to announce a change of mind. If no one objects, the decision becomes official.

An alternative approach is the legal document known as "Termination of Parental Rights" (TPR). In this case, the mother applies for a time slot in county court. (Crowded schedules may mean a delay of four to six weeks.) The mother and her parents sign preliminary papers beforehand.

The father has a lesser role. He will receive a summons, by registered mail, to attend the court session. He is not required to do so, however, and usually does not unless he objects to the adoption.

The court session itself lasts just a few minutes. The judge will ask for assurance from the mother that she agrees to the adoption of her own free will without pressure. When these matters are clarified, the mother's rights cease on that day, and the child becomes eligible for adoption. (As previously mentioned, procedures may vary somewhat in different states.)

• *Independent adoption*—At this writing, many states permit independent adoption, although different restrictions apply which are undergoing constant revision. That means that no agency serves as intermediary. The adoption is arranged by a third party, such as a doctor or lawyer. This person establishes contact between the expectant mother and a couple who want to adopt a child. Terms are arranged; they can be quite flexible. In some cases, the couple pays for the woman's medical care and related costs during pregnancy. Sometimes the parties establish a personal relationship: the adoptive couple may attend childbirth class and delivery with the mother. Adoptive parents receive full custody after the child's birth, but sometimes the birth mother can maintain ties with the child and the adoptive parents through letters, audio- and video-taped messages, exchange of pictures, etc.

Adoptive couples like the fact that this method can be finalized much more quickly than with the formal process of working with an agency. Since adoptive couples are making private arrangements, they may face less stringent criteria such as age, income, and health. As a general rule, the time and paperwork involved are less than when working with an agency.

There are drawbacks, however. Adoptive couples may not be screened as carefully as they would be by an agency; this could give incompetent or abusive people access to children. Similarly, there may be inadequate analysis of the adoptive home environment itself and the adoptive parents' goals for the child. And even in the best of situations, the more intimate relationship between adoptive and birth parents may backfire. Finally, should the ties between birth and adoptive parents become too strong, children could suffer the anxiety of not knowing whom to call their "real" parents.

• *Open vs. closed: a difference in philosophy*—Elements or degrees of open and closed adoptions can occur in both agency and independent systems.

Closed adoptions mean that the records containing identifying information are sealed. The parties know little about each other. The child, throughout life, has little opportunity to learn about the birth parents. This is the most conservative approach. It secures confidentiality, but it is contested by many who urge greater accessibility of the files.

There are many levels of open adoption which can be found in both agency and independent procedures. This option is increasingly popular. Unwed mothers appreciate the "human touch" it offers. Since open adoption holds the possibility of ongoing relationships with the child, it reduces the stress of releasing one's flesh and blood to another's care.

Nontraditional approaches to adoption pose distinct challenges. Above all, it is essential to serve the child's interests—to enable the development of a secure identity.

No one model, procedure, or type of adoption can meet the needs and concerns of everyone. This is why we are fortunate today that most states allow diversity and experimentation. We are constantly finding new ways to make adoptions more loving and humane, and we are a spiritually richer society because of this effort. [1]

Questions Concerning Adoption

Of course, not all cases go so smoothly. There can be many complicating factors. The following questions are samples of the issues that might arise to make the involvement of an attorney or social worker desirable. Answers should be used only as a springboard for your own discussion and solutions:

What will my child know about me?

Open adoptions are flexible; it's up to the biological parents to make decisions about this with the adoptive parents. Agency adoptions, however, tend to give fewer options, but the choices may be more clear-cut and easy to follow.

Having the mother write a letter to the child has proved workable. In it she describes her interests and background, and she can explain why she chose to place the child for adoption and why she chose this particular couple as parents. Have her include a description of herself: height, weight, coloring, hobbies.

Writing a letter can help a mother break ties with the child. It provides an important way to say "goodbye" and bring a sense of responsible closure to the transaction. The letter also will give a child a sense of roots and identity. Depending on your state's laws, there may be limits on the amount of identifiable information that may be included (such as mother's name and place of employment or school).

The adoptive parents must decide when and how to share this letter with the child. Some adoption counselors urge parents to discuss adoption with their children at an early age, to remove the mystery and anxiety that can surround such an event. Introduce the subject naturally, with answers adjusted to the child's level of comprehension, much the same as a discussion of sex. Over time, talks can become more detailed. A gradual building process is preferable to the sudden announcement: "You're adopted."

Adoptive parents appreciate information about their child's biological parents. It can help them when the child begins to show musical ability, for example, or has difficulty learning how to read. If health problems run in the birth parents' families, or if substance abuse had a role in the pregnancy, this information will be of great value as adoptive parents seek the best care for the child.

What will the adoptive parents and I know about each other?

Generally, it's the right of the birth mother to select the couple who will adopt her child.

Couples who wish to adopt a child need to make themselves known and, in a sense, "sell" themselves as prospective parents. There are long lists of couples who want to adopt white infants. (Waiting time is considerably less, though, for minority, mixed-race, handicapped, and older children.) Prospective adoptive couples who prefer the open method might place newspaper advertisements and have their names circulated among doctors and lawyers. Couples who choose the agency approach have a more straightforward assignment. They submit biographical information and have their home environment analyzed by licensed social workers. This information goes on file and they are alerted when a child of their preference becomes available. Couples who want to adopt are asked about their age, income, education, personalities, hobbies, religious convictions, and other children in the family. The couple also state their views on money management, discipline, educational opportunities for the adoptive child, etc.

When a couple is chosen to adopt a child, they also learn about the mother in general terms. Sometimes this information comes from the mother herself, or the agency supplies it in her behalf.

What are the mother's rights?

The birth mother is the central character in this story. Even when placing her child for adoption, she has considerable authority. For example, she can forbid the father, even if he admits paternity and wants to help, from having any role during her pregnancy.

If the mother wishes to rear her child alone, she may name the father to secure his financial support. If he admits paternity, he is responsible for costs until the child is 18 years old. If he denies paternity, the woman can legally compel him to have a blood test. The test is not foolproof (it tends to confirm who is *not* the father), but its results generally are binding. It cannot be performed until the child is six months old. But if a man is identified as the father, he may have to pay on a retroactive basis those costs the mother already has incurred.

What if the child has birth defects?

Mental or physical handicaps can radically change the picture of adoption.

Agencies usually have a provision to release prospective adopters if the child is born with defects. Open adoptions, by their more informal nature, are not as structured. No one likes to contemplate this problem, but all parties would be wise to discuss contingency plans should it happen.

A mother still can terminate her rights to a such a child. In this case, the agency or state tends to become guardian of the child. Alternatively, the mother may retain her rights and place the child in foster care, until another adoptive couple is found. This may take considerable time. During the waiting period, the mother may have to pay some of the costs of foster care.

The Father's Role

Many young men who are caught up in a crisis pregnancy question their relationship to the baby. Sometimes, they want to avoid responsibility. In other cases, especially if the girl has multiple boyfriends, there may be genuine doubt. Given this ambiguity, men have several possible levels of involvement.

A 1972 Supreme Court decision requires a man to be notified that he might be the father of a child who is being placed for adoption. The man has the right to contest the adoption, in which case the process may be delayed or stopped. If the man is or was married to the birth mother, or if they lived together, the man's consent may be required for adoption to take place. In other cases, no consent is necessary.

The man may claim he is not the father. In such a case, blood testing can help determine paternity. Testing does not prove paternity, but it can establish who is *not* the father. The process can take several weeks. One such test, the Human Leukocyte Antigen test, is sophisticated and costly, but the results are highly accurate. The test can be done through many blood banks and laboratories specializing in paternity testing. The results are admissible as court evidence in many states.

For an adoption to proceed, the woman is encouraged to name an *alleged father* of the child. This man need not admit paternity, but he is asked to sign documents that release his *potential rights*. If the woman names more than one man, each alleged father must release his potential rights.

Many men do not wish even this degree of involvement. In this case, the alleged father simply need not attend the court session that ends the mother's rights. The judge will interpret a failure to appear as indication that the man has waived his rights, and the adoption can be completed. In other cases, it may be impossible even to locate the alleged father. He may have left the community, or he may refuse any contact with the mother. (Also, the mother may be unsure whom to name as the father of her child, or she may be afraid to identify the individual.) In this case, the adoption agency publishes a notice in a local paper.

The notice states that the woman has given birth to a child. The mother's name is published and so is the child's. The notice will request the father, named or not, to come forward. Typically, the notice runs in the paper for three weeks. A ten-day waiting period must follow. If, by that time, the father has made no contact, the adoption agency may petition a judge to waive the father's rights.

The name of the alleged father does not appear on the child's birth certificate without his permission. The mother has the right to name the child, and in most cases she assigns her last name to the child. (Both names, of course, may be changed by the adoptive parents.)

Should a man admit paternity, he has the first right to parent the child once the mother releases her rights.

Agencies and Programs to Support the Single Mother

Unfortunately, many hospitals routinely conduct abortions, and many other public agencies encourage abortion as an acceptable option for unplanned pregnancies. This does not

110

mean that a woman with a crisis pregnancy shouldn't use the other services offered by these agencies, but you may need to support her resolve to carry the baby to term if she seeks their help and comes under their influence. The following are some of the government and community agencies offering resources to the single mother. Since these agencies vary widely from state to state, a good place to begin to find help is to contact your State Department of Human Services. This department should be able to supply the telephone numbers for specific agencies.

• *Aid for Families with Dependent Children*—AFDC is a federal cash grant program for women whose salary and liquid assets fall under a certain minimum level. Monthly allowance is determined by the size of the family. Medicaid and food stamps are other federal resources distributed through local welfare offices that help provide necessities.

• *Women, Infants and Children*—WIC is a service that is similar to food stamps. Distribution takes place at the Public Health Department. Eligible mothers receives vouchers for basic food and baby needs, such as cheese, milk, and formula.

• *Crisis hotlines*—Counseling by telephone is a helpful, anonymous way to cope with stress. Some hotlines are case-specific, with applications for rape, pregnancy, loss of a loved one. Other hotlines, are designed for more general situations, such as anger or frustration with parenting. But most will accept a call from anyone in crisis. If the person who answers is not equipped to handle the caller's needs, he or she can "hear out" the caller and refer her to other experts who can give more detailed assistance.

Most hotlines are operated by nonprofit social service agencies. The majority are staffed by trained volunteers. The overall purpose of a hotline is to let the caller vent emotions; find a sympathetic, anonymous listener; and dispense useful information. Hotlines do not offer ongoing, customized therapy but can refer callers to other resources.

Many hotlines operate 24 hours a day, every day of the year. This is of particular value for people who become depressed or anxious about their problems outside of business hours—nights, weekends, holidays. The crisis hotline should only be the first step in seeking treatment and not an end unto itself.

• *United Way*—This organization has been serving community needs since the 1880s. Its statement of purpose reads: "To increase the organized capacity of people to care for one another." United Way is an "umbrella" organization, with a wide array of separate agencies under its sponsorship. The number and type of member agencies will vary among communities, but they typically cover needs such as housing, medical referrals, and counseling. Call the United Way headquarters in your community to get a listing of what is available.

• *High school guidance officers/college counselors*—A teen mother may be concerned only with the next few months. You will do a major service if you encourage her to think of her future, especially her education.

There are many options. Some communities have special schools (or special classes within a public school) for teen mothers. Others have on-campus day-care facilities. It may be possible for a mother to take a reduced course load and stretch out the time needed to finish her degree; or she may complete her schooling by correspondence, night class, or special testing. Tutoring programs may be available in the after-school hours to help her build skills. If a mother is motivated to further her education, most schools will be delighted to work with her. Check with local foundations to see if educational grants and scholarships are available.

• *Hospital personnel*—Most hospitals have a chaplain, information officer, or social worker. These people can provide a listing of medical services within the hospital itself; they also may refer you to specific physicians who treat individuals in a crisis pregnancy. These resource people can help with information about billing and insurance. Many hospitals and doctors may be willing to waive fees or extend the payment schedule to accommodate a mother on a tight budget.

• *Public Health Nurse*—This person can offer similar types of information, assisting in scheduling medical appointments, designing nutritious meals, and making sure all medications are taken and instructions are followed.

• *County Social Service*—Consult this agency for advice on low-cost housing, day-care for children, and social workers who can counsel teen mothers. Your local district attorney's office may have attorneys available to assist in establishing paternity and in collecting child support. Many lawyers offer reduced rates for low-income cases. Some associations of lawyers even specialize in serving the needs of poorer people.

• *Service clubs*—Rotary, Kiwanis, and Jaycees are part of the life of most communities. Members are business leaders with a sincere desire to help. A number of clubs have grants to help individuals in need. Contact them when you need help for a specific person or to set up a program of ongoing assistance. Some service club members may be able to arrange a part-time job at which a teen mother could work to enhance her self-respect, financial independence, and development of marketable skills.

• *Pastors' associations*—Naturally, you can go to individual churches. This may be especially effective if the woman you're helping is a member of the congregation or if you need limited financial aid which could come from a benevolent fund.

The way to reach a larger audience, though, is to work through pastoral associations. You could make a presentation at their regular meeting. Tell the members about the incidence of unwed pregnancy in your community; show what is being done to serve these women and which needs remain unaddressed. Challenge their support through local missions, women's groups, and youth organizations in the church.

• *Maternity homes*—A few generations ago, many counties had homes for "unwed mothers." In that day, great stigma was attached to being a single parent. Since even mainstream women did not work outside the home, it was very difficult for single mothers to support themselves and their children.

Maternity homes went out of fashion when it became socially acceptable for women to rear their children alone. About the same time, federal and state programs offered financial assistance and county/local funds were redirected.

Today, maternity homes are making a comeback. Often they are sponsored by a church or private agency. They provide low-cost shelter, meals, and the benefits of group support and modern counseling. In this kind of positive environment, it's possible for women to set new direction for their lives.

One of the dictionary definitions of *crisis* is "a turning point for better or worse." The challenge to make this crisis a turning point for better does not lie with the young mother alone. As Christians, this responsibility is shared.

Perhaps the best news about crisis pregnancy is that people are getting involved. Through churches and agencies and as concerned individuals, Christians are taking a stand. They are denouncing abortion. And they are offering constructive solutions to help teen mothers turn their lives around. As God leads, I hope you will be moved to take a stand. There is a special enrichment that comes when you know you have had an impact on someone's life. The opportunities for service are all around, limited only by your imagination.

Introduction
1. Karen Pittman and Gina Adams, *Teenage Pregnancy: An Advocate's Guide to the Numbers* (Washington, DC: Children's Defense Fund, January/March 1988), p. 4.

Chapter One
1. Elizabeth Stark, "Young, Innocent and Pregnant," *Psychology Today*, October, 1986, pp. 28-30.
2. Claudia Wallis, "Children Having Children," *Time*, December 9, 1985, pp. 79-90.
3. Stark, "Young, Innocent and Pregnant."
4. Ibid.
5. Wallis, "Children Having Children."
6. Ibid.
7. Marion Wright Edelman, *Families in Peril: An Agenda for Social Change* (Cambridge, MA: Harvard University Press, 1987).
8. Virginia Satir, *Peoplemaking* (Palo Alto, CA: Science and Behavior Books).
9. *Harvard Education Letter*, May, 1987.
10. Curt J. Young, *Least of These* (Chicago: Moody Press, 1983), p. 158.
11. Wallis, "Children Having Children."
12. Ibid.

Chapter Four
1. Beverly O'Brien, *Mom . . . I'm Pregnant* (Wheaton, IL: Tyndale House Publishers, 1982), pp. 24, 25.
2. Linda Roggow and Carolyn Owen, *Handbook for Pregnant Teens* (Grand Rapids, MI: Zondervan, 1984), p. 42
3. Ibid., p. 115

Chapter Five
1. *Teen Sex Survey in the Evangelical Church*, Executive Summary Report, P.O. Box 811, Salem, OH 44460, p. 3.
2. "Life Lines: What You Can Do About Abortion," *Christopher News Notes*, 12 E. 48th St., New York, NY 10017, No. 301, p. 2.
3. Ibid.

Chapter Six
1. *The Bantam Medical Dictionary* (New York: Bantam Books, 1982).
2. Curt J. Young, *The Least of These* (Chicago: Moody Press, 1983), p. 19.
3. Ibid. p. 115, 116.
4. Michael Gorman, *Abortion and the Early Church* (Downers Grove, IL: InterVarsity Press, 1982).
5. Ibid., p. 33.
6. Ibid., p. 34.
7. Ibid., p. 49.
8. Tertullian, *Apology*, p. 9.
9. Gorman, p. 59.
10. Ibid., p. 66.
11. Young, p. 50.
12. Ronald L. Koteskey, "Growing Up Too Late, Too Soon," *Christianity Today,* March 13, 1981, pp. 24-28.

Chapter Seven
1. Douglas R. Donnelly, *A Guide to Adoption* (Pomona, CA: Focus on the Family, 1988), p. 15.

BIBLIOGRAPHY

Brandt, Patricia, with Jackson, Dave. *Just Me and the Kids.* Elgin, IL: David C. Cook Publishing Co., 1985.

Part of the Family Ministries series on family life stages, this 13-session course addresses the particular needs of single parents, many of whom have experienced a crisis pregnancy and face the prospect of raising their child alone. The course helps single parents deal with loss and separation, anger and guilt; accept themselves and their present situation; develop realistic parenting goals; build and maintain family identity within the context of biblical family functions; and utilize the resources of the extended and church family, among other important topics.

Garton, Jean Staker. *Who Broke the Baby?* Minneapolis, MN: Bethany Fellowship, Inc., 1979.

Having successfully reared a family, Jean Garton wanted time to pursue her own goals, so it was a bitter shock when she learned she was pregnant at age 40. At the time, abortion on demand was illegal; Garton had the baby, but she joined a group seeking to have the laws changed. Eager to build the strongest argument possible, she examined law, medicine, history, and philosophy. But as she delved further, she found to her surprise that, in the words of C.S. Lewis, "I was carried kicking and screaming" to the pro-life stand "by the sheer weight of the evidence." This book traces the progress of her thinking. Written with elegant simplicity, Garton's book examines the leading pro-abortion slogans. Although it charts some of the most deceptive thinking of our time, the message of this book is hopeful.

Gorman, Michael J. *Abortion and the Early Church: Christian, Jewish and Pagan Attitudes in the Greco-Roman World.* Downers Grove, IL: InterVarsity Press, 1982.

Abortion seems so much an issue of the twentieth century that few people even think to analyze how the first Christians viewed

117

this procedure. Surprisingly, abortion was a pressing concern from the early days of the Church, and Gorman provides a comprehensive view of how the Christians grappled with it 2,000 years ago. This book is helpful in providing a lay person's definition of scholarly terms, while at the same time including thorough notes and references for people who want to do more in-depth research. Some readers may disagree with Gorman's conclusion, which links the Christian perspective on pregnancy with that concerning nuclear arms control. But few will dispute his call for "a consistent affirmation of life," a clear reminder that no issue exists in a vacuum.

Johnson, Lissa Halls. *Just Like Ice Cream*. Palm Springs, CA: Ronald N. Haynes Pub., 1982.

This highly readable account of Julie, a high school girl who gets pregnant, covers her relationship with her boyfriend, parents, and best girlfriend. The title comes from a ploy used by the boy: "What if you never had any ice cream until you were 25. Say your parents 'protected' you and said it wasn't good for you. Say you finally had some and found out you loved it. Wouldn't you be disappointed that you hadn't started enjoying it sooner in life?"

Of course, Julie learns that sex and ice cream are very different. She also finds value in life, the meaning of salvation, and forgiveness. *Just Like Ice Cream* is never stuffy—enjoyable reading for you and adolescents.

McDowell, Josh. *How to Help Your Child Say "No" to Sexual Pressure*. Waco, TX: Word Books, 1987.

Part of McDowell's "Why Wait?" campaign, this book equips parents with practical "how to say no" principles to share with their teenagers, as well as creative preventative measures for parents of preteens. This realistic and sensitive book is a helpful resource for parents who want their children to know that waiting until marriage is the best choice they can make about sex.

McDowell, Josh. *Teens Speak Out: "What I Wish My Parents Knew About My Sexuality."* San Bernardino, CA: Here's Life Publishers, 1987.

Another book in the "Why Wait?" series, *Teens Speak Out* is an important resource for parents, pastors, and youth workers, who need to understand the pressures teens face and listen to their gut-level struggles in their own words. Some chapters are compiled from questionnaires, letters, and essays written by teens themselves on parents, peers, pressure, and premarital sex. Other helpful chapters are entitled, "51 Reasons for Sex," "47 Reasons to Wait," and "37 Ways to Say No."

McDowell, Josh. *Why Wait? What You Need to Know About the Teen Sexuality Crisis.* San Bernardino, CA: Here's Life Publishers, 1987.

Another in the "Why Wait?" series, this book describes the crisis in teen sexuality, explores in depth the reason Christian youth are having premarital sex, expands on the physical, spiritual, emotional, and relational reasons to wait until marriage for physical intimacy, and gives parents and those who work with youth useful ways to help them cope with the pressure.

O'Brien, Beverly. *Mom . . . I'm Pregnant.* Wheaton, IL: Tyndale House Publishers, 1985.

This book intertwines a compelling personal story with practical advice on a wide range of issues related to crisis pregnancy. When O'Brien's 19-year-old daughter spoke the words that form the title, the author records the gamut of emotions she and her family felt: anger, fear, worry, resentment. But she emphasizes that no situation is beyond hope. Slowly, and with many difficulties, the family learned how to cope with the situation. O'Brien recounts the step-by-step process with which her family structured the problem so that it became manageable. The book offers common-sense information about legal matters, assistance from social agencies and hospitals. O'Brien says the best help for a pregnant teen and her family has never changed: the constant love of God.

Powell, John. *Abortion: The Silent Holocaust.* Allen, TX: Argus, 1981.

As the title of his book suggests, Powell sees a chilling parallel between the Nazi policy of death and abortion in America today. He gives enough background into Nazi Germany to satisfy readers who are not familiar with that epoch, but he also draws conclusions that will engage the attention of experts. Powell makes ample use of quotations from both the popular media and medical, governmental, and philosophical writings. He provides thorough citations, so readers can use the original sources as a springboard for additional research. Powell's work is particularly valuable for showing how seemingly remote philosophical discussions shape daily events, which can result in life or death for its citizens. The book also is an articulate synthesis of works from many leading Christian thinkers. Best of all, Powell's style is not academic. He conveys a truly conversational tone on paper.

Roggow, Linda, and Owens, Carolyn. *Handbook for Pregnant Teenagers*. Grand Rapids, MI: Zondervan, 1984.

This is an exceptionally practical guide for young women in a crisis pregnancy. Roggow is a social worker and Owens is a writer. The product of their collaboration is a comprehensive yet easy-to-understand road map of stages to expect when coping with a problem pregnancy. Roggow and Owens cover all the major issues: health care for mother and child, decision-making skills, finances, and relationships with the child's father and both sets of grandparents. The book has a worksheet approach, posing questions and leaving space for a teenager to write in her answers. In some cases, this borders on the simplistic. Yet that is also one of the book's strengths: providing a bottom-line assessment. Perhaps the greatest value of the book is its calm tone. Roggow and Owens make it clear that problem pregnancy is not an easy situation, but their methodical approach shows how the situation can be handled.

Schaeffer, Francis A. *The Great Evangelical Disaster*. Westchester, IL: Crossway Books, 1984.

Schaeffer wrote this book just before his death, saying it contains "perhaps the most important statement I have ever written." A major theme of this book is the danger of compromise: Nothing must interfere in our relationship with God, and no amount of pressure must sway our behavior from the clear standards God sets forth in the Bible. Many people endorse abortion not because they are committed to it, but because it *seems* the easiest or most practical alternative. Schaeffer insists that the only safe course is to obey God's commands, even when they appear impossible or out of touch with conventional wisdom. This is because the world's definition of what is right and good always changes or gives way to pressure. God's values are permanent. Implicit in Schaeffer's writing is a call to activism. If we stand still, we will see first our society and then our churches erode into spiritual wasteland. This book bears a persuasive Schaeffer touch: Christian analysis of the popular media. It is not light reading, but its important message makes the extra concentration worthwhile.

Waters, Ethel. *His Eye Is on the Sparrow.* New York: Doubleday & Co., Inc., 1950.
Books abound that describe crisis pregnancy from the perspective of medicine, law, and theology. There are many painful accounts of the women who have gone through such a crisis and a small but growing literature on the experiences of men at these times. There are very few books, however, that give the point of view of the truly innocent party: the child. Ethel Waters fills that void in her powerful, sad, and funny autobiography. She was conceived when her mother, age 12, was raped at knife-point in a ghetto. Today, many people would say that such a tragedy can best be handled only by abortion. Waters's life refutes that claim. Left to run wild in the slums, she developed herself into a world-famous actress and musician. Today she is properly remembered for expressing the human dignity of blacks. But we also should value her as proof that even the most "unwanted" person, who seems to have the lowest "quality of life," is a full member of the human race.

Weddle, Linda Massey. *I'm Not Laughing Anymore.* Lincoln, NE: Back to the Bible, 1984.
A fictional account of a crisis pregnancy, written from the viewpoint of a teenage mother, this book covers 15 months in the life of her family. Weddle reveals how unwed pregnancy can happen to the families who expect it least. The heroine of this story, a Christian, meets her boyfriend at church; many of their dates center on youth group activities. But none of this is enough to prevent her from engaging in sexual relations or prepare her for the hard decisions that follow. Teenagers who can identify with the white, middle-class characters will benefit from reading this book. Counselors will find this book of perhaps even greater value, since it offers especially clear insight into the values and interests of young adults as well as the social politics of a family

that is not well-prepared to deal with a crisis.

Wheat, Ed, M.D. *Love Life*. Grand Rapids, MI: Zondervan, 1980.
Wheat is a physician whose writing combines accurate psychological and medical information with solid Biblical insight. *Love Life* is a best-case scenario. It outlines God's principles for a rewarding marriage. Mutual submission, the ways to seek one another's best interest, and methods to keep love alive are highlights of the book. An especially poignant chapter is called "How to Save Your Marriage Alone." It gives the Christian response when one partner is determined to abuse or end the relationship. The message is clear: With God, all things are possible. Many people going through a crisis pregnancy need to hear those words. The truth behind them may seem removed from daily life, but this message can give an attainable ideal, a goal they can achieve. Wheat's discussion of sexuality and the differing needs of women and men can help readers set a new direction in their lives.

Willke, Dr. and Mrs. J. C. *Abortion: Questions and Answers*. Cincinnati, OH: Hayes Publishing, 1985.
The Willkes are internationally recognized for their expertise in the disciplines of human sexuality and human rights as related to the abortion issue. Their commentary program, "Pro-life Perspective," is an institution on Christian radio broadcasts. The format of this book is easy to read, organized on a thematic basis: history, fetal development, how abortions are performed, difficult cases, etc. The book draws upon medical literature that gives solid documentation, but the Willkes are careful to explain unfamiliar terms and to delete unnecessary, confusing material. They also quote effectively from the pro-choice literature, showing its internal contradictions and hidden agendas, many of which are not known to the general public. Writing style is geared for the lay person who does not have a technical background.

Young, Curt J. *The Least of These*. Chicago: Moody Press, 1983.
Young is executive director of the Christian Action Council, which works with a nationwide network of Crisis Pregnancy

Centers. His book gives the "big picture" of problem pregnancies. He includes case studies, national statistics, and biblical analysis. Young shows that abortion is not the answer—for either individuals or society at large. Instead, Young offers numerous, viable alternatives for both mother and child. Young concludes with practical advice on how individual Christians and churches can take an activist position. He covers worship services, prayer support, and legal means of protest, showing there is a place for all who are willing to take a stand.

Other Resources

American Citizens Concerned for Life
P.O. Box 179
4000 Leslee Curve
Excelsior, MN 55331
(612) 474-0885

Christian Action Council
701 West Broad Street
Suite 405
Falls Church, VA 22046
(703) 237-2100

Focus on the Family
P.O. Box 500
Pomona, CA 91769
(714) 620-8500

Life Cycle Books
P.O. Box 792
Lewiston, NY 14092-0792
(416) 690-5860